BLACKS, MEDICAL SCHOOLS,
AND SOCIETY

Blacks, Medical Schools, and Society

James L. Curtis, M.D.

Foreword by John Z. Bowers, M.D.

Ann Arbor
The University of Michigan Press

DEDICATED TO THE MEMORY OF
FRANKLIN C. MCLEAN, M.D.

Founder of National Medical Fellowships, Inc.,
and leader in the desegregation of
medical educational opportunity

33990

Foreword

The past three years have seen a dramatic change in the position of blacks in medical education. Three years ago they sought opportunities to study medicine; today black students are being sought in a nationwide talent hunt by the medical schools.

During this three-year period, the number of blacks entering the study of medicine has tripled—from 266 in 1968 to 697 in 1970—and there is every indication that this rate of increase will continue for a period despite intensive competition for black talent from other education fields and from industry. The sharp increase of blacks going into medicine has resulted from a range of recruitment programs stimulated by faculty members who are conscious of the unfortunate disparity between the eleven percent of black citizens in the United States and the two percent of black physicians. A comparable disparity applies in other professions with the probable exception of the clergy. Primarily, the recruitment programs are aimed at junior and senior high school students and college students. However, other efforts include summer fellowships in medical research laboratories; supplementary educational programs at the college level focused on the premedical sciences and communication skills; an adjustment of the admissions process in relation to the educational background of black applicants; and specialized guidance and counseling services. Although definitive statistics are not yet available, the impression is that the academic mortality and morbidity rates among black students is not significantly greater than that of the total body of medical students. Attention is now turning to other minority groups such as Puerto Ricans, Mexican-Americans and American Indians.

In his introduction to *Negroes and Medicine* (1958), Franklin McLean, who may be described as the father of the modern movement to integrate blacks in medicine, stated, "The problems of Negro medical students have shifted dramatically and consistently in recent years." He went on to point out that the number of predominantly white medical schools enrolling black students had increased from twenty to forty-eight. Today the shift is even more dramatic and essentially every medical school is enrolling black medical students.

As James L. Curtis points out in this book, the first eight schools to enroll blacks were in the North, and for some of us there was mounting concern that this would strip the South of its potential talent for medicine. It is heartening, therefore, that southern schools are now joining actively in the identification and preparation of blacks for the study of medicine.

Although the major efforts to prepare and recruit more blacks for the study of medicine are no more than five years old, important lessons have already been learned that deserve full reporting and analysis—in a sense, a living history. Dr. Curtis is uniquely qualified to write such a document. His twenty-five years of experience began with one of the earliest awards from the National Medical Fellowships, Inc., then known as Provident Medical Associates, to support his residency training in psychiatry and psychoanalysis. Deeply concerned about the severe shortage of black physicians, James Curtis led a program of the Provident Clinical

Society of Brooklyn, a branch of the National Medical Association, to identify and give educational support to junior high school students in the Bedford-Stuyvesant section. The striking success of this pioneering program, recounted in detail here, was only one of the factors that brought Dr. Curtis national recognition as a leader in the movement to expand black medical education.

When Cornell Medical College decided to enlarge its program for the recruitment of minority group students, Dr. Curtis was a natural choice for the position of director of the program. Thus our author has the unique qualifications of having started as the director of a talent-recruitment program at the high school level and of having now added a rich experience in college-level recruitment in his role as counselor in a medical school.

Dr. Curtis buttresses the objective and analytical presentation of his personal experiences in the field with a historical review that is urgently needed today. Also included is a valuable compilation of the essential statistics relating to the paucity of Negroes in medicine.

Dr. Curtis's book is an important reference source for all individuals who are concerned not only with the education of our black citizens but other minority groups as well.

JOHN Z. BOWERS, M.D.
President, Josiah Macy, Jr., Foundation

Preface

Writing now as a "black" physician in 1970, I would only a year ago have preferred to be called "Negro"; and going back to 1946 when I graduated from the University of Michigan Medical School, I would have felt equally at ease at being called "colored." Current confusion, among blacks as well as among whites, over the correctness of this or that racial label has neither aided nor impeded certain basic and positive changes which are occurring in American higher education, particularly in the area of medical education. Without attracting much public attention, the system of undergraduate medical education has begun to get rid of the color barrier, as a direct result of conscious plans and programs to bring greater numbers of blacks into the predominantly white medical schools. This development should be more widely known, not only because of its obvious fairness, but because it brings us closer to a day when all physicians, irrespective of color, will be able to treat all patients, irrespective of color, with the same high standard of excellence and care. A single, color-blind system and standard of health education and health care is a first step in the more difficult transition toward a system which will be blind to social class difference as well.

Medical education up to now has been a tightly segregated system in which the two predominantly black medical schools have graduated an estimated eighty-three percent of the six thousand black physicians in the country, while the ninety-nine predominantly white schools with superior resources in faculty, facilities, and predominantly public money have graduated only token numbers of black doctors through the years. The pattern has changed decisively within the past two years: Counting all first-year medical students entering all the one hundred and one medical schools in the fall of 1969, for the first time more than half of them were attending one of the ninety-nine predominantly white schools. This expansion, both in quality and quantity of medical educational opportunity for blacks, is a direct contribution to improving the public health. It will also ensure that blacks will participate at leadership levels with the other future leaders of American medicine who will be forced to develop a much-improved system of medical care. Predictably there are powerful forces working for and working against this favorable movement and change.

In this book an attempt will be made to describe the present situation and to describe the development and decline of the segregated pattern; problems which remain to be resolved in increasing the pool of qualified black high school graduates, and a description of specific efforts to do this; and a description of a specific attempt to strengthen the premedical preparation of black premedical students, presenting material from the special summer program of collaboration with Hampton Institute and several other colleges and universities and the Cornell University Medical College. The impact of these changes on the white and the black medical schools, and continuing unresolved debate on the meaning and significance of this new effort will also be explored. The summer projects were crucial in strengthening Cornell's participation with other leading schools in a deliberate expansion of admissions opportunities to blacks and other minority groups.

It is a matter of some urgency that opportunities for medical careers be made known to black and to other under-represented minority-group students, for they read and hear little to give them cause for hope that they can look forward to any significant and major leadership role in the mainstream of American institutional life. It is a matter of vital importance that black students be encouraged to assume that all career opportunities will continue to expand for them, that they should not assume that it is "unrealistic" for a black to aspire to this or that subspecialty, or that they can only look forward to becoming general practitioners in ghettoes, whether they would find that to their liking or not.

Naturally I am recalling some of my own uncertainty in making a decision as to whether or not I should specialize in psychiatry and psychoanalysis after I had graduated from medical school and completed my internship almost twenty-five years ago. In that day opportunities for internships and residencies were few and far between. There were in fact only eight Negro psychiatrists in the whole country. Just about that time, a small number of leaders in the field of psychiatry let it be known that their programs of residency training were open to Negro applicants, and that there would be every reason for them to anticipate successful careers in the field. There are now about three hundred black psychiatrists, a third of them fully certified, with a wide range of successful careers in public and private practice, teaching, research, and administration, most of them in racially integrated settings.

Not only in psychiatry, but in other medical specialties, postgraduate training opportunities for Negroes began to open up in the 1950's, a decade or so earlier than in the area of undergraduate medical education. The late Dr. Franklin C. McLean founded the National Medical Fellowships, Inc., to help develop such training opportunities and to provide the able Negro postgraduate trainee with financial aid to allow him to pursue additional training. I am one of the specialists who received a fellowship grant under that program. Most of us look eagerly to the day when the overall opportunity gap between black and white Americans will be closed, so that there will be no further need for special programs to provide an equal start for all. In the meantime, the task before us all is to work together toward becoming a single community rather than the separate and unequal antagonistic nations we have been for so long.

Acknowledgments are especially due the Macy Foundation for supporting Cornell's summer research fellowship programs with a $93,000 grant for the three-year period 1969–1971. Many thanks are due Dr. John Deitrick, former Dean of Cornell University Medical College, and Dr. Jerome Holland, former President of Hampton, who planned the Hampton collaboration. We are indebted to Cornell's current Dean, Dr. J. Robert Buchanan; Associate Dean Lawrence W. Hanlon; and to Dr. E. Hugh Luckey, President of the New York Hospital–Cornell Medical Center; all of whom gave helpful support in many forms. I am also grateful to many other faculty members, especially Dr. Walter Riker and Dr. Walsh McDermott; and to Cornell medical students, especially Robert Robinson, Jeffrey Gingold, Timothy Lane, James Cohen, and John Mitchell.

I acknowledge the tremendous support received from my colleagues of the Provident Clinical Society of Brooklyn whose Scholarship Committee, of which I was chairman, spent the past six years prior to my coming to Cornell in directing our volunteer work with promising minority group high school students who might be interested in medical careers. Thanks are due the professional colleagues who accepted my invitation to take part in Seminars on Careers in Medicine, which brought a personal note to the students' increasing awareness of the broad range of opportunities in the medical field, as well as major problems and challenges in the various specialties.

We are also much indebted to those who made materials available which were indispensable to the preparation of this manuscript: AAMC staff members, Dr. Davis Johnson and Mr. Dennis Dove; Dr. Dietrich C. Reitzes for permission to use material from his book, *Negroes in Medicine;* Mrs. Hilde Reitzes of National Medical Fellowships, Inc.; and Miss Maxine Bleich of the Macy Foundation; and the *Journal of The American Medical Association.*

It is a pleasure to express my deep appreciation to Dr. John Z. Bowers, President of the Josiah Macy, Jr., Foundation, who encouraged and supported this work, and who kindly consented to write the Foreword for the book. Also I wish to thank Mr. Marvin Raeburn, Director of Public Information for the Medical College, who gave me important advice and assistance in planning the book. Many thanks and much appreciation are also due Mrs. Mary Land, who provided skillful secretarial assistance.

James L. Curtis, M.D.

Cornell University Medical College
New York City

Contents

I

Historical Perspectives

Race and History

The anthropologist Franz Boas was a leader in the drive to do away with myths of racial superiority and inferiority which caused such serious problems both here and abroad.[1] He made the following points: There are no pure races; the children of immigrants to the U.S. undergo, in time, changes in body type which set them off from their parents; much of what we consider to be innate or hereditary is really culturally acquired; and no racial group has any sound basis for claims of superiority over other groups, even though such claims have been made with great regularity whenever two groups live together in a mutually dependent, dominant-submissive relationship, with strong motives to remain apart. Specifically with regard to the Negro, Boas pointed out that while their contribution to scientific cultural advance has been relatively slight during the last two hundred years since the Industrial Revolution has been under way, the Negro undoubtedly played a great role in the very beginning and crucial stages of human civilization.

V. Gordon Childe has pointed out that most of our historical distortions come about from the fact that we try to read too much significance into events which occur within a given country, among a few of its rulers and key people only, within a few hundred years.[2] All our written documents take us back only about five thousand years. By including the period of human prehistory, we must consider the last five hundred thousand years. This would take in the time during which men became definitely differentiated from the more apelike hominids, and learned to fashion the first crude tools from stone and to make a fire. The first major rush of discoveries or inventions came in Egypt and Babylonia between 5000 and 3000 B.C., and were: artificial irrigation, the plow, use of animal power, sailing boats, wheeled vehicles, orchard husbandry, fermentation, production and use of copper and bronze and iron, the use of bricks, the arch, glazing, the seal, the solar calendar, writing, and numerical notation.

Negro historians (see Franklin,[3] Bennett[4]) have summarized the Negro contribution to the civilization of ancient Egypt. It seems certain that the ancient Egyptians represented a fusion of several racial groups: the Mediterranean Causasians, the Semitic nomads from the East, and the brown and black tribes from Nubia and from ancient Ethiopia. Representative members from all these racial stocks are prominent among all the social classes, including their priesthood and nobility. Nefertari, wife of Ahmose I, co-founder of the Eighteenth Dynasty, was Negro. Ethiopian ascendancy was marked in the first millennium before Christ, the Ethiopian domination was complete for more than a hundred years until the Assyrian conquest of Egypt in 670 B.C. As Asian and then Christian influences strengthened in Egypt and in Ethiopia during the first millennium after Christ, it is thought that some of these darker people may have migrated to the western coast of Africa, judging from what appear to be definite Egyptian influences in such West African cultures as Yoruba and Benin.

Most is known about the ancient West African
kingdoms of Ghana, Mali, and Songhai which flourished
in the period 700 until about 1600 A.D. When the Arabs
set out to convert the world to Islam in about the eighth
century of our era, they moved eastward to India, and
westward through North Africa, up into Southern
Europe, and down into the Western African Sudan.
They encountered strong feudal kingdoms in West
Africa, which had tight control over large numbers of
people with great standing armies, and with control
over established trading caravan routes. The Muslim
success was not militarily decisive, but their cultural
influence was tremendous. There was a vast expansion
in trans-Sahara caravan trade, with the West Africans
sending gold and slaves, rubber and ivory in exchange
for textiles, brass, and salt. Several large and important
trading centers were established, and became the home
of important universities such as Timbuktu, Gao,
Walata, and Jenne. Scholars and students learned
not only the religion of Islam, but also about law, liter-
ature, the sciences, and medicine. There was considerable intermarriage, and some amount of conversion
to Mohammedanism. These West African nations were
culturally on a par with, or more strongly effective than,
most European nations during the same time. All this
ended with the opening up of Africa to the slave trade,
with the coming of Christianity and the era of modern
European history.

As Herbert M. Morais has pointed out, the myths,
taboos, and prejudices which have worked against
Negroes as health professionals and as patients are
deeply rooted in the American past.[6] He goes on to say,
" . . . The story of Jim Crow in medicine and health is a
story worth telling, especially now as a burgeoning and
deepening Negro freedom movement focuses attention
not only on jobs, votes, schools and housing, but also on

medical care and health. It is a story of . . . professional talents wasted and of a people's health undermined." The papers by M. O. Bousefield[11] and Leonard Johnson[12] are useful as brief historical summaries of Negroes in American medicine.

In this brief survey of some of these major historical phases, we shall note the persistence of a few dominant themes: Is the black man inferior mentally? Can he be integrated into the same society with whites, or should he be segregated or exiled?

We shall also note what Gunnar Myrdal emphasized, that white Americans have always suffered a dilemma of conscience concerning the Negro, have been always unable wholly to accept or to reject him.[5] As Eli Ginsberg and Alfred S. Eichner remark, "The white majority was able to hold the Negro minority in bondage and then in subservience for almost three and a half centuries by institutional arrangements that were relatively easy to introduce and maintain."[7] As they mention, World War I and then World War II brought about an expansion of American industry whose manpower needs pulled Negro unskilled and unused labor from the agricultural South into unionized industries in the North and West, into communities which provided better health and social and legal services, and a better education for their children. Earlier in this country Negroes advanced only accidentally, as it suited the political or economic needs of conflicting whites; only now is the Negro on the threshold of power and influence that will enable him to achieve his full citizenship.

Early American Period (1619–1812)

When the first group of nineteen Negroes were brought to Jamestown, Virginia, they were treated somewhat along the lines of white indentured servants. There did not exist a legal or social status for a slave, but this status was gradually evolved before 1700. By that time, while whites could come into a colony and contract out their services for a given number of years, after which they would be free, Negroes were kept in permanent servitude unless they were able to purchase their freedom or were set free by their masters. Moreover, their children were also automatically enslaved; they had no civil, political, legal, or property rights.

Massachusetts was the first state to give a legal status to slavery in 1641, followed by Connecticut in 1650, Virginia in 1661, Maryland in 1663, New York and New Jersey in 1664, South Carolina in 1682, Rhode Island and Pennsylvania in 1700, North Carolina in 1715, and Georgia in 1750.[4] That there was a sense of unease about the institution is shown from the fact that Vermont abolished slavery in 1777, followed by Massachusetts and New Hampshire in 1783. Pennsylvania provided for gradual emancipation in 1780; Connecticut and Rhode Island barred slavery in 1784. New York provided gradual emancipation in 1799, followed by New Jersey in 1804. Negroes had at first come into the country slowly; by 1700 there were only 20,000, but by 1790 there were 550,000 slaves in the country, about one-fifth of the entire American population. Slave labor in the South, where the principal crops were tobacco, indigo, and rice; and slave-trading by New Englanders made Negro slavery the keystone of the nation's economy.

Medicine of that day was primitive, and at the time of the Revolution there were 3,500 practitioners of medicine in all the colonies, of whom 3,100 were apprentice-trained and only 400 were university-educated physicians. The first African physician in the colonies is thought to have been Lucas Santomee Peters, a Dutch-educated physician who was voted a special grant for his service in 1667 by the New York colony where he practiced. The Negro slave known as Cesar published a remedy for snakebite in the *Massachusetts Magazine* in

1792, the first medical publication by a Negro. It is known that there were more than a few self-taught or partly trained healers like him with a following.

James Derham, born in 1762 in Philadelphia, was probably the best-trained and most successful Negro practitioner of that era. Though slaves were not supposed to be taught to read or write, he was given this instruction in the family where he grew up. He was then sold or given to a Dr. John Kearsley, Jr., one of the leading American physicians, whom he assisted and from whom he learned to compound medicines. Kearsley was a Tory and was executed during the War, following which Derham became the property of a Dr. George West, a surgeon with the 16th British Regiment. At the close of the War, West sold Derham to Dr. Robert Dove of New Orleans, who also utilized him as a physician's assistant. Dove allowed Derham to purchase his freedom and set up practice in New Orleans, where he became a considerable success. Benjamin Rush and other leading abolitionists often cited Derham as proof that blacks were potentially as capable as whites, a controversy which 'was well established in the Revolutionary Period.

By far the most important contribution to medicine of the colonial era came from a slave named Onesimus who taught his master, the very influential Cotton Mather, a technique of smallpox inoculation which had originated in Africa. This reference[8] was first called to my attention by Frances Hamilton, Cornell University Medical College's interlibrary loan librarian, who assembled an exhibit on January 26, 1970, covering approximately three hundred years of the contribution of blacks to American medicine. Cotton Mather was one of the religious leaders who insisted that slave masters should instruct their slaves in the gospel and allow them to become converted and members of church congregations, insisting that they remained like brutish heathens as a result of their masters' neglect. The Church of England in England maintained constant pressure, with little effect, on the colonists to christianize and convert the heathen slaves, who were thought to be the spiritual equals of their masters. But as Jordan has analyzed the situation, church membership would have carried with it very often the right to vote and to hold office, to testify in court, and to be entitled to other rights which separated slaves from free white men.[9]

In 1706 Cotton Mather was given a young male slave, whom he named Onesimus, and whom he considered intelligent. When asked whether he had ever had smallpox, the young man described the method by which he had been inoculated in Africa, showed Mather the scar, and claimed that it was a general practice among his tribe, that they were given a mild case of the disease as a protection against subsequent attack. Since smallpox epidemics were a periodic scourge, Mather became convinced that the method should be tried experimentally in this country, and despite considerable opposition and controversy it was tried with success from the time of the 1721 smallpox epidemic throughout the Revolutionary War period. We should recall that Jenner's published work in England in 1798 came decades later, and that Waterhouse only reintroduced the method to the U.S. in 1800. While many of Mather's opponents derided him for believing that a slave would have anything important to teach, it is worth noting that Mather had allies, among them Benjamin Franklin, who helped spread this method of prophylaxis against smallpox to Philadelphia. Furthermore, as Jordan mentions, in all the controversy and debate nobody claimed that "a medical procedure which would work with Negroes might not work with white men."

But the central difficulty for Americans in this colonial period was that they did not know what to do with free Negroes, who made up about a tenth of the black

population in the Revolutionary decade. Increasingly
the pressure was to freeze them in a status as close to
slavery as possible, and to leave considerable distance between their status and that of free whites. Thomas Jefferson, who believed he had kindly feelings for Negroes,
led the school of thought that Negroes were innately inferior physically and mentally to whites, and that free
Negroes would never be accepted as equal citizens by
whites, but should be resettled in some faraway
country. Not in a single colony did free Negroes enjoy
the full rights to jobs, education, voting, and other privileges. In the South it was feared that they would spur
slave revolts, a fear which increased with the Gabriel
Conspiracy of 1800, and with the news that the slaves
of Haiti who revolted in 1791 had proclaimed themselves and their country free in 1804. In the North work-
ing-class whites feared that free Negroes would depress
wages, and upperclass whites feared that they would increase the crime rates and the relief rolls. However, the
number of free Negroes began to increase; antislavery
sentiment and colonization enthusiasm among whites
increased also in the period around 1800, because the
system of southern plantation agriculture was beginning to become unprofitable. This situation changed
dramatically after 1810, by which time Eli Whitney's
invention of the cotton gin had suddenly made cotton
a fabulously profitable crop. Slavery became immediately more popular than ever, and was increasingly
justified by racist doctrine.

Pre-Civil War and
the Rise of Jim Crow (1812–1944)

The American Colonization Society was founded in
1816 with the support of many of the most prominent
Americans, in the North as well as the South, with the
aim of sending free Negroes from the U.S. to the west

coast of Africa. In fact a tiny settlement was established there and came to be known as Liberia, but the tremendous cost of this venture made it clear that it was wishful thinking to suppose that this kind of venture would resolve the Negro-white American problem. Free Negroes immediately denounced colonization as an unjust move to deprive them of their rights to full citizenship to which they felt entitled, many of them having fought in the Revolutionary army and navy, and many others realizing the contribution that unpaid black labor had made to the nation's growth. Ironically, however, the American Colonization Society was the first major source of encouragement for the training of Negro doctors for the purpose of going to Africa, or to some black nation such as Haiti, to care for their brethren. The abolitionists were of course also interested in promoting educational opportunities for Negroes, but it is well to bear in mind that even some who wanted to abolish slavery were still persuaded that Negroes should emigrate to another country.

While there were probably no more than a dozen or so Negroes who were admitted to any American institution of higher learning for any period of time before then, it was not until 1828 that Jones at Amherst and Russworm at Bowdoin became the first of their race to receive the Bachelor's Degree from an American college. In 1847 David J. Peck became the first of his race to receive the M.D. from an American medical school, Rush Medical College. In 1849 Bowdoin College (which then had a medical school) conferred M.D. degrees on John V. DeGrasse and Thomas J. White. Of both of them it has been said that their schooling had been for the purpose of preparing them for medical missionary services in Liberia, but they refused to carry out that expectation. DeGrasse had several additional years of medical study in Europe, and on his return to this

country he became a highly successful practitioner. He
was the first Negro member of a medical society (Boston Medical Society and the Massachusetts State Medical Society), and later during the Civil War he was the
first Negro surgeon to be commissioned by the United
States Army. Academic requirements for the M.D. degree were minimal in that day, consisting mainly of attending lectures for periods of six months in each of two
years. By 1860 at least nine medical schools had admitted one or several Negroes: Bowdoin, the Medical
School of the University of New York, the Caselton
Medical School in Vermont, the Berkshire Medical
School in Massachusetts, the Rush Medical School in
Chicago, the Eclectic Medical School in Philadelphia,
the Homeopathic College of Cleveland, the American
Medical College, and the Medical School of Harvard
University.

The rigidity of the color barrier was such that the
first few professionally trained Negro physicians went
abroad. Perhaps the best known of these men was Dr.
James McCune Smith, born into a free Negro family of
means, who received his early schooling at the New
York African Free School but was then unable to gain
admission to college despite his obvious ability. He was
matriculated at the University of Glasgow, where he
received his B.A. degree in 1835, an M.A. in 1836, and
the M.D. in 1837. He returned to New York where he
set up an extensive practice with much success, but
he gradually began to devote more of his time to the
abolitionist movement as a writer and orator. He pas-
sionately opposed the colonization movement, and he
appeared in public debate against the eminent Senator
John C. Calhoun from South Carolina, who was a leading protagonist of colonization and of pro-slavery myths
of Negro inferiority. This is not to imply that there was
not a small number of Negroes, even among those prom-

inent in the abolitionist movement, like Sojourner Truth, who were sympathetic toward colonization and racial separatism because they felt that America could not accept blacks as equal.

An apprentice-trained physician, a man of considerable ability, was Dr. Martin R. Delany, born in 1812 in Virginia. His family moved during his boyhood to Pennsylvania where he received good schooling along with other children in their small town. By the age of nineteen he had moved to Pittsburgh, where he was busy as a writer and speaker for the abolitionist cause and at the same time began serving an apprenticeship with a leading physician. He served three such apprenticeships (at least one being a requirement for medical school admission of that day), but he was turned down by all the four schools to which he applied: The University of Pennsylvania, Jefferson Medical College, and the Medical Schools of Albany and Geneva in New York. Later he applied, along with two other Negro candidates, to Harvard, and all three of them were admitted to the 1850–51 class, notwithstanding the fact that a pro-slavery faction of students passed a resolution condemning their acceptance as an attempt at "amalgamation of the races."[6] Delany did not complete his studies at Harvard, but returned to Pittsburgh to practice medicine and to continue his work against slavery. Within a few years he and a small group, including another Negro physician, Dr. David J. Peck mentioned previously, tried to set up a separate Negro state in Nicaragua, but it failed and they returned to the U.S. In 1859 he went on a geographical mission to explore the Niger River valley; and although he lectured and wrote on this subject, he did not make an actual attempt to resettle in Africa. During the Civil War Delany played a leading role in convincing President Lincoln of the wisdom of using Negro troops. Delany himself recruited them, and was commissioned and served as a regular Major in the infantry; he did not serve in the medical corps of the army.

The eight Negro physicians who did serve in the medical corps were all university-trained. It was a scandal of which some note was made, however, that the 37,300 Negro soldiers who fought in the Union Army suffered a casualty rate at least a third higher than that of the white troops, that the War Department was reluctant to assign Negro or white physicians to these Negro troops, and that Negro physicians did not receive any more pay than Negro enlisted men received.[6] It is also worth mentioning at this point that of the five thousand Negroes who participated in the Revolutionary War, most fought in racially integrated units.[4] This is another barometer of the gradually increasing racial polarization. By 1840 there were approximately four hundred thousand free Negroes in the United States (about thirteen percent of all Negroes), and some of them had substantial means.

As C. Vann Woodward has explained, the rigid segregationist policies which have come to be known as "Jim Crow" were invented in the pre-Civil War era in the North to serve the purpose of maintaining white supremacy and Negro subordination in communities containing whites and free Negroes.[10] With the end of the Civil War in 1865 and with the Negro no longer a slave but free, the South imported the Jim Crow policies from the North as a replacement for their former master-slave control system. Southern slavery had not required nor even allowed for any great amount of physical separation between the races. The hard line on racial separatism only gradually gained control in the South in the decades following Reconstruction from 1870 to about 1900. It became increasingly prevalent during the first two to three decades of the 1900's, by which time segregation was accepted as a longstanding and ancient part of the American way of life, North and South.

The wretched conditions among the masses of freedmen in Washington, D.C., demanded immediate action of some kind after the Civil War, for there were over 22,000 unemployed Negroes there, and a like number who were patients in government hospitals. Faced with the massive need for emergency health, education, job-placement, and welfare services, it was clear that a university which would be open to all persons without regard to color was an important need. Howard University was opened in 1866 and its medical school opened in 1868 as an attempt to meet some of these urgent needs. Only seven Negro physicians practiced in Washington, D.C., then. The Howard University Medical College opened with eight students, one of whom was white, and five teachers, one of whom was Negro. Tuition was low and classes at first were held from 3:30 p.m. until 10:00 p.m. in order to allow poor students to earn a livelihood by holding federal jobs on which the workday ended at 3:30 p.m. The Howard faculty was highly regarded by the American Medical Association, which itself had been founded in 1847. Several of the white faculty also were faculty members at Georgetown University, and all were dedicated to the cause of the Negro. The very able Negro faculty member, Dr. Alexander T. Augusta, through lack of admission success in this country, had obtained his medical education at Trinity Medical College in Toronto, Canada. On returning to the U.S., he had served in the Civil War as surgeon, first with the rank of Major and later Lieutenant Colonel. He was a faculty member with the title of Demonstrator of Anatomy, while all the other faculty, no doubt with more standard and prestigious medical school origins, had the title of Professor in their various fields. From the first, the school was known to be well run. It was also dedicated to the rights of women to enjoy medical educational opportunities. In 1877 on a motion brought by the Jefferson Medical College, the Howard delegation was not seated, because at Howard men and women were taught in the same classes. A measure of the success of the school is shown by the fact that by the year 1890 Howard had graduated 253 students, including 15 women, students who had come from all the states—especially the North—and from several countries in Africa and the British West Indies.[6]

The other medical school for Negroes established during this era was Meharry Medical College, founded in 1866 as part of the Central Tennessee College. While it was supported by the Freedmen's Aid Society, it did not receive full governmental support and subsidy as did Howard's medical school. Meharry Medical School actually did not go into operation until 1876, with less than a dozen students and with two white faculty members. Unlike Howard, this school was established expressly for Negroes, and primarily for Negroes from southern states who had only marginal preparation to pursue medical studies. In fact, it was not until 1923 that Meharry was accredited as a Grade-A medical school. However, it should be mentioned that Meharry had graduated 102 students by 1890.[6]

Three Negro faculty members of the Howard Medical College made application for membership in the local AMA branch in Washington, D.C., in 1869. On being turned down, they and their white supporters attempted to bring their application for membership to the Annual Convention of the AMA in 1870. They failed to overturn the action of the local medical society, and the fight went on at annual meetings for the next few years until it was abandoned in 1884, the attempted resolution being that whites and Negroes would form a separate and independent, racially integrated, local medical society. The Negroes who had been unsuccessful in their application for membership were not satisfied with that arrangement, and by the year 1895 an all-Negro medical society had been formed.

As a result of the racially exclusivist policies of the AMA, a great number of local all-Negro medical societies were formed during the 1880's. This set of actions was an unfortunate accommodation to the infamous Hayes-Tilden Compromise of 1877 in which the Republican, Rutherford B. Hayes, became President of the U.S. by a single electoral vote, presumably in exchange for a northern concession to the South. All federal troops stationed in the South to safeguard the freedmen's rights were withdrawn in the interest of national white solidarity and national unification. As C. Vann Woodward has observed, there was not only a collapse of white liberalism, North and South, which might have protected the cause of Negro freedom and full citizenship; but Negro leadership faltered, perhaps unwittingly, with Booker T. Washington's admonition in the Atlanta Compromise Address of 1895 that the races should be separate, blacks should be humble and submissive, and not much interested in political or social equality.[10] In these same decades the appeal of the Populists was being diminished by determined efforts, especially in the South, to drive a permanent wedge between poor whites and poor blacks and to bring about a progressive disfranchisement of blacks.

W. E. B. Dubois, the Negro leader who firmly opposed Booker T. Washington, and whose efforts finally led to the formation of the National Association for the Advancement of Colored People, was dedicated to the full integration of Negroes into every facet of American life and leadership. The separatists, white and black, prevailed and the development of two separate nations gradually increased from the latter decades of the last century into the first few decades of the 1900's. Six additional all-black medical schools were formed after Howard and Meharry, and these were abandoned only when the Flexner Report of 1910 began to exert reformist pressure on all American medical educational institutions to move into the new era of scientific medical practice or go out of business. But these schools, which operated from 1882 or thereabouts until after the reaction to the Flexner Report, had graduated a total of about one thousand black students, of whom nearly half had passed state boards, and who continued to function as practitioners even after their schools' demise.

Not all Negroes gave up their attempt to avail themselves of the best possible medical education of their day. The case of Dr. Francis Mossell is illustrative. He was accepted on his application to the University of Pennsylvania in 1876. He was asked to sit behind a screen in the classroom, which he refused to do. At first no other student would sit next to him, but shortly he made friends, and on graduating high in his class in 1882 he had many supporters of his application for membership in the Philadelphia Medical Society, and he was successful after a brief struggle. Returning to Philadelphia after an additional brief period of study in England, he was compelled by the deprivation of medical care and medical training opportunities for blacks in that city to establish a segregated hospital for Negro patients, where they could receive first-rate care and where young Negro doctors and nurses would be able to receive training and staff privileges.[6]

A progression of U.S. Supreme Court decisions from 1873 to 1898 had led to the entrenchment of the "separate but equal" doctrine which guaranteed inferior treatment for Negroes. Gradually it became the rule that Negroes and whites were cared for only in separate wards of general hospitals, if Negroes received

admission at all. There was sometimes a legal requirement that Negro patients could be cared for only by
Negro nurses, and that no white nurse could care for a
Negro male patient. Patients were to be cared for in separate hospitals for the mentally ill; separate or segregated facilities were to be provided in nursery homes
and also in orphanages, in institutions for the deaf,
blind, and dumb, and in penal institutions and ceme-
teries.[10] While World War I was fought "to make the
world safe for democracy," presumably including our
more than 360,000 Negro troops and their relatives,
there was a series of dangerous race riots in the last
six months of 1919, North and South, as an expression
of white reaction against any real change of attitude. It
should be mentioned that 356 Negro officers were commissioned in the U.S. Medical Corps during World War
I, and they operated a segregated hospital for the 92nd
Division which served overseas.[6] Of these, only one held
the rank of major.[11] In 1920, there was in the United
States a total of about 3,855 Negro physicians, most of
whom had graduated from Howard and Meharry. This
number, as an absolute number of Negro physicians in
the country, was not to change for more than twenty
years.

During World War II, we may note for purposes
of comparison that as of 1943 there were 582,861 Negroes in the army. There were over 4,000 commissioned
officers, representing certainly a vast expansion in the
number of officers as contrasted to any earlier war; but
the total number of commissioned medical officers was
only 395 for the Medical Corps, 67 in the Dental Corps,
and 202 in the Nurses' Corps. While Negroes ran a much
bigger segregated hospital in World War II than the
one in World War I, there were only one Negro medical
officer with the rank of lieutenant colonel and ten
majors.

It was beginning to be clear that the development of Negro medical manpower had just about come to the end of the road under the system of segregated medical education. In fact, the total yearly production of black physicians was running just a few under the one hundred a year who died.[11] It had become clear to Cobb[13] and to the NAACP, as well as to others, that Howard and Meharry alone could not solve this problem; that there was no need for a third, all-Negro medical school; and that no segregated scheme of any kind would be a satisfactory substitute for doing away with the dual system of medical education and health care.

Cobb pointed to such facts as these: Howard and Meharry were forced to accept applicants whose aptitude test ratings were regularly below the national mean because they came from states with inferior segregated primary, secondary, and college school systems. Many came from southern states which spent on the average twelve times more for the education of whites than for Negroes. The graduates of Howard and Meharry had disproportionately high rates of failure in passing state board examinations to practice medicine. After these examinations were passed, they had only restricted opportunities for postgraduate medical education. As of 1947, of the ninety-three Negro physicians who were specialists, slightly more than half were graduates from predominantly white schools which had graduated only about fifteen percent of all Negro physicians. Going on, he said that fifty years ago there might have been no alternative except to expand segregated medical school facilities, but not now. "The present indication is for Howard and Meharry to open their doors to more white students and for the other 75 medical schools to admit such qualified applicants as might appear. It is only through a program of intelligent integration that the health needs of the Negro, which are inseparable from those of the general population, can be met."[14]

Integration Struggle Continued (1944–1970)

The Great Depression had an undeniably liberalizing effect on the American political atmosphere, and the racial groups began to move into the same political parties and labor unions—all of which was given added impetus by World War II which had as a major motive the necessity of freeing the world of racist terrorism. The post-war, cold war tensions between East and West, as well as the rise of the underdeveloped non-white nations with their increasing claims to a role in world affairs, also provided a basis of growing support for the long struggle for first-class citizenship for American blacks. From the late 1940's up to now a progression of Supreme Court decisions have attempted to undo the restricting separatist rulings from the turn of the century, which had in effect denied Negroes the full protection of legalized society. But we are still in a period of great turbulence, with a continuing preoccupation with the ancient issues of integration or separation. It is still debated whether Negroes are inferior in intellectual capacity, and whether it is possible for the two races to live together as equals in one democratic nation. It may well be that ancient Egypt can give us cause for hope in the possibility of a multiracial, but strong and united, community.

In ancient Egyptian history, the Old Kingdom (2700–2200 B.C.) has been called the Age of the Pyramids, and it is during that time that they achieved their greatest in art and architecture. The pyramid designed by Imhotep (2700 B.C.) is the oldest known stone structure in the world. Imhotep, in addition to being a great architect, was also a priest and physician who gradually came to be considered a demigod following his death, and was deified as the god of medicine during the rule of the Ptolemies. We are especially interested in Imhotep, because some of the likenesses of him reveal that he had Negroid features. The name Imhotep means "He who cometh in peace."

In 1956, an organization was formed under the leadership of W. Montague Cobb, editor of the *Journal of the National Medical Association* as well as professor and head of the Department of Anatomy of Howard University Medical College. This organization was called The Imhotep National Conference on Hospital Integration, possibly reflecting the new style of linking American blacks with their African and even Egyptian ancestors, in a new assertion of black pride. This was not intended, however, to be a racially separate movement at all; quite the opposite, for it was set up with a three-fold purpose: to press for laws to put an end to segregated hospital services, to promote lawsuits to prevent public funds from supporting the construction or operation of segregated services, and to advise governmental bureaus and administrations on means to remove racially discriminatory practices and patterns. The sponsoring organizations for this conference were the National Medical Association, the Medico-Chirurgical Society of the District of Columbia, and the National Association for the Advancement of Colored People. A date was set in March 1957 for the first Imhotep Conference to be held in Washington, D.C. Invitations were extended to the American Medical Association, the American Hospital Association and other leading hospital agencies to send representatives to this conference to discuss action to eliminate segregation and discrimination from hospital services. The invited organizations named above did not send representatives. Nor was there a response from other invited organizations such as the American Nurses' Association, the National Health Council, the United States Health Service, the

American Protestant Hospital Association, and the Catholic Hospital Association.[6]

Year after year for the next seven years, annual Imhotep Conferences for Hospital Integration were held in various cities. Support gradually developed, not only from Negroes, but increasingly from whites who were active in civil rights and labor, as well as the enlightened leadership of a number of communities, which gradually opened their doors to Negroes as patients and as staff members. But even as late as 1963 at the Seventh Imhotep National Conference, Cobb remarked on the continued refusal of representatives of the chief, organized medical groups to take part in these meetings. Not until 1964 did the American Hospital Association issue a statement to the effect that medical and hospital care should be made available to all without qualification of any kind.

Later in 1964 the Secretary of Health, Education and Welfare, Anthony J. Celebrezze, convened a meeting in Washington, D.C., to discuss means of eliminating racial bias in hospitals by voluntary action. This meeting was attended by blacks and whites, including representatives from medicine, dentistry, nursing, and hospitals, as well as other high governmental officials. Even before that meeting, the hospitals under religious auspices had become increasingly responsive to pressures to admit patients and to appoint staff members without regard to color. By 1966 considerable progress had been made, and it has been summarized as follows (in *The Negro Handbook*'s section on "Negroes in Medicine"):[15] The federal government outlawed segregation and discrimination in governmental health facilities, meaning that Negro patients and staff were accepted in hospitals operated by the Armed Forces, the Public Health Service, and the Veterans Administration; all of these changes were underway during the 1950's. Secondly, when Congress extended the Hill-Burton Act in

1964, under which states would be provided with financial support to build hospitals, nursing homes, and rehabilitation centers, they struck out the words allowing them to create so-called "separate-but-equal" facilities, since these had been shown to be but a cover for denial of equal access to good health care and had also been declared unconstitutional. Lastly, the 1964 Civil Rights Act's Title VI assured that no federal funds could go to any program from which anybody was excluded for reasons of race, color, or national origin. An Office of Equal Health Opportunity was set up in the Justice Department's Civil Rights Division to check hospitals to see whether or not their practices were indeed obeying the law.

As was pointed out by James G. Haughton[16], who is black and who is First Deputy Administrator of the New York City Health Services Administration, "The functions of the Federal Office of Equal Health Opportunity have recently been transferred to the office of the Secretary of H.E.W. This step has been hailed by some who have made no secret of their opposition to Title VI of the Civil Rights Act of 1964." He went on to urge militant watchfulness to assure that the public's rights to unsegregated health care be maintained, since there already exist explicit government guarantees that all should have access to health care regardless of color or race, and equal opportunity for professional education, and for the formulation of health policy as well. In that article, Haughton leaves no doubt in anybody's mind that there can be no separate or piecemeal approach to safeguarding the health of American blacks as a separate project, because up to now they have suffered as have other Americans from the lack of federal governmental acceptance of responsibility for the health needs of our citizens. Starting, however, with the Social Security Act of 1935, which offered federal grants to states providing health care for certain categories of needy persons, and with the 1965 amendments commonly known as Medicare and Medicaid which greatly expanded the financing of health care, it is inevitable that the government will also be required to play an active role in creating an effective and responsible system of health care and of maintaining standards for services purchased.

Neither black nor white Americans have enjoyed a high level of health care, nor has the level of care been reliably good or acceptable even for middle-class Americans who could afford good care. This is partly because the medical schools have put almost exclusive emphasis and status on the importance of research and the obtaining of new knowledge, rather than on matters of delivery of health care. It is for this reason that the National Medical Association, almost all of whose members are Negro, is able to approach matters of health policy from a point of view different from the perspective of the American Medical Association, whose members by and large represent the more privileged American middle class. Certainly, as is well known, the NMA provided earlier and important support for Medicare at a time when it was vigorously opposed by the AMA. But the matter is not so simple. Gunnar Myrdal observed only a few decades ago that Negro physicians in very great numbers are among the strongest opponents of anything that resembles socialized medicine, or even standard public health services, or the expansion of municipal hospital services.[5] The reasons cited were plausible enough: Negro physicians, because of prejudiced attitudes, had difficulty attracting black or white patients; they had less chance of being as well trained or maintaining high-level skills; they were excluded from hospital appointments; they were also not hired as staff members to run public health services or municipal hospitals or other facilities. The few patients they had were therefore jealously guarded, because there was no room for the Negro physician in the other systems. It is easy to see from this perspective that the general point of view of Negro physicians in matters of health policy for all the people, black or white, could only become more responsive and sensitive as the relaxation in the color barrier allowed them to become a part of the general health manpower situation.

There are some who say that the members of NMA should maintain themselves as much as possible as an all-black organization, because only in this way can they be sure of remaining faithful to the health needs of American blacks. In the preceding paragraph I have shown that the system is far too complex to be understandably analyzed, managed, or predicted on the basis of skin color or race alone. My own inclination is to hasten the day when the NMA will have no further need to exist as a separate organization of black doctors, but will be able to exert even greater influence by energetic involvement in AMA organizational activities, leading the profession at large into a more responsible and responsive role in terms of the health care needs of all Americans. For years the AMA in effect excluded many Negroes from joining their principal professional organization, inasmuch as one could not be a member of the national body without holding membership in the local and state AMA chapters. Until recently of course this excluded blacks in the South. Local and state initiative in dropping this practice was to be the approved solution, with many localities lagging and the national AMA refusing to force open membership. In 1964 it was something of a victory that the AMA voted itself as being unalterably opposed to such exclusion, and called upon component societies to exert every effort to end such racial exclusion. Each year attempts are still made to tighten up the resolution in one way or another, although Negro physicians who have been denied membership are probably becoming harder and harder to find.

We have now, however, almost come full circle to a time when white physicians who wanted to become members of the (black) National Medical Association during the 1960's found that their applications were received in lukewarm fashion. During the civil rights protest marches and demonstrations in the early 1960's, the Medical Committee for Human Rights, a racially integrated organization, provided medical care for civil rights workers and others in southern deprived areas. The MCHR at times found that their presence was not welcomed, if not actually resented, by NMA representatives. It has not yet been clarified that whites are desired as members of NMA; quite usually they are only tolerated, and only rarely do they hold important offices in local branches. A comfortable format has not been found for black and white physicians to function easily, with shared roles as leaders and followers, in the major medical organizations. The problem has perhaps been best resolved by small, progressive-liberal medical groups, but these are only of limited influence.

The National Dental Association, the organization of black dentists, stated as recently as 1965 that in eleven of the southern states the American Dental Association will only rarely accept Negro members, by specific exclusionary clauses in their bylaws or by unwritten agreement. While the American Dental Association has since 1962 had the power to punish those state societies which discriminate in this way, that Association has not exercised any disciplinary action.

From 1951 to 1968, as Morais[6] has remarked, the American Nurses Association made steady progress toward integrationist goals in the nursing profession. This followed the decision made by the ANA to accept all the members and primary organizational aims and purposes of the National Association of Colored Graduate Nurses, an organization set up in 1908. The NACGN voted unanimously in 1950 for dissolution the following year, even though (or because) it was a strong organization with over 11,000 black members whom it had served well for over forty years. There was no real need for two separate organizations, the nurses reasoned, and since that time Negro nurses have served on the national board of directors, as well as on some state boards of the ANA. Equal employment opportunities are sought, official registries and placement services are used by the single organization, and Negro nurses are increasingly found in all facilities as well as among faculty and administration of schools of nursing. This does not mean that the fight for equality has been won, for there are still instances of job discrimination or racial salary differentials, of segregated nursing schools or token integration in some other nursing schools, and too few examples of Negro nurses with significant roles in policy-making.

Summary

Myths asserting the intellectual inferiority of Negroes are not supported by a knowledge of African history, nor by awareness of the history of blacks in the United States. First slavery and then an inferior castelike status has been the lot of all but a few fortunate individuals who broke free of these restraints. Even before the Civil War a number of Negroes had been well trained and had practiced medicine in the best tradition of their time.

Following the Civil War and in line with relegation of freed slaves to second-class citizenship roles, Negro medical schools and medical societies began to come into existence in response to a need to provide health services to freedmen and the fact that training opportunities still only existed for a token few.

The weaker Negro medical schools were forced to close, leaving only the two strongest ones, Howard and Meharry, after 1920. The number of Negro physicians remained constant at just under four thousand in the decades between World War I and World War II, at which time it became apparent that unless expansion of medical educational opportunity occurred, there would barely be a replacement of those who died or retired.

Since the 1950's, with the move of the mass of the Negro population, about half now live outside the South and the majority of blacks live in large cities. This has improved their access to health, education and employment resources, and has allowed them to develop sufficient social and political power to determine at least in part their future development.

The rise of the civil rights movement, the lessening of socially sanctioned color barriers, the continued shortage of physicians and other health personnel provide additional basis for programs to encourage potentially able black youngsters to pursue medical careers. Despite a promising advance from the Depression era until after World War II, within very recent years, racist separatist attitudes and philosophies, so much a part of the American past, have worked against the formation of effective coalitions among Negroes, the poor, and other disadvantaged groups.

In the next chapter we shall see how effectively such coalition of groups has been in the recent past. In the chapters to follow we shall explore various means to increase the pool of qualified Negro aspirants for medical career opportunities.

II

The Current National Trend
in Medical Education for Negroes

Medical Manpower Pool

School desegregation seems almost a lost cause, some fifteen years after the Supreme Court declared against it. Its opponents in the South, who continue to frustrate it by every legal, procedural, and political means are joined by those in the North who preach a doctrine of despair that residentially segregated housing patterns will ever allow any meaningful school integration to occur. Even in formerly liberal circles, it is becoming fashionable to announce that integration is a dead issue, not desirable even if attainable, and feeble attempts to rationalize this stand are made. Fortunately this air of gloom relates itself primarily to school desegregation at elementary and high school levels. At the levels of college, graduate, and professional schools an important amount of desegregation has taken place within the past few years. Certainly, in one area of American higher education, in medical education as a whole, a clearly new trend is developing.

Black Americans make up 11.03% of the slightly more than two hundred million Americans; they constitute 6.0% of the almost five million undergraduate college enrollment (just under half of them being enrolled

in Negro colleges); in the fall of 1969 they made up
2.75% of the medical school student body enrollment
of almost 38,000; they had 2.2% of the 230,000 or so
practicing physicians; and similarly 2.4% of the 83,000
or so practicing dentists. These data, recently prepared
by Mr. Dennis Dove and other members of the Association of American Medical Colleges staff, are presented
here as Table I.[1] The situation is one of graphic under-
representation, even though it is not so dramatic for
blacks as for the numerically smaller groups of American Indians and Spanish-surnamed Americans. We have
a challenging opportunity as a nation to resolve this
problem at this time. Only within the past few years
has there developed a consensus that we do have a
physician shortage in this country; only recently is medical care coming to be considered a right, to be provided
by public funds if necessary; and now it is becoming
apparent that our needs for medical manpower will
never be met until we begin to provide a higher level of
education than ever to greater numbers of educationally
underprivileged Americans from minority groups.

There is cause for hope in the next few years. In
data from Table II, taken from the same source, we
have an analysis of the number of black college freshmen in the country, giving their percentage of the nationwide total, and whether they were attending predominantly black or predominantly white colleges. It
can be seen that there a promising increase in total numbers and percentages, and that undergraduate black
college students are increasingly attending predominantly white schools rather than the weaker, segregated, black colleges in the South, which up until very
recently provided the chief source of higher education
even for Negroes from the North. It is pertinent to note
here that the same percentage of black freshmen express
an interest in pursuing a career in medicine or dentistry
as of white freshmen (approximately four percent).

TABLE I

Statement of Problem

	Population Size 1960		Under-graduate Enrollment Fall 1968		Medical School Enrollment Fall 1969		Practicing Physicians 1960		Practicing Dentists 1960	
	Number	%	Number	%	Number	%	Number	%	Number	%
Total	201.2 million		4,819,819		37,756		230,307		83,198	
Black Americans	22.2 million	11.03	287,053	6.0	1,042	2.75	5,038	2.2	1,998	2
American Indians	523,591	2.30	29,493	0.6	18	0.04	25	0.01	NA	NA
Spanish Surnamed	3,464,999*	15.46*	90,879	1.9	92	0.24	NA	NA	NA	NA

NA = Not Available

*In five Southwestern states.

Sources: 1. U.S. Department of Health, Education and Welfare/Office of Civil Rights "Undergraduate Enrollment by Ethnic Group in Federally Funded Institutions of Higher Education, Fall 1968" (OCR-201-69)

2. Association of American Medical Colleges, Fall 1969 Enrollment Questionnaire

3. 1960 U.S. Census

TABLE II

Trends in Black College
Freshman Enrollment 1966–1969

Year	Total Freshman Enrollment	Black Freshman Enrollment		Freshman Enrollment at the Predominantly Black Colleges	
		Number	%	Number	%
1966	1,163,123	58,156	5.0	NA	NA
1967	1,359,883	58,474	4.3	15,841	27.0
1968	1,472,929	85,429	5.8	38,729	45.3
1969	1,637,831	98,269	6.0	39,465	40.1

Source: American Council on Education
National Norms for Entering College Freshmen, 1966, 1967, 1968, 1969.

The crucial importance of desegregating the under-graduate collegiate preparation for medicine, so far as Negroes are concerned, is seen from the fact that on a nationwide basis all first-year medical school students for at least twenty years have come from less than eight hundred colleges and universities.[2] Much less than half of these schools supplied more than seventy-five per-cent of the entire entering class of medical students. Looking at the fifteen-year trend, one can say that three hundred and fifty of these leading colleges, or about half of them, supplied ninety percent of medical school freshmen; that as few as one hundred and seventy-five, or a quarter of them, supplied seventy-five percent of all medical freshmen. In fact, "Twenty-five schools, comprising only three percent of the undergraduate institutions supplying one or more medical students, provided an average of twenty-eight percent of the four entering freshman classes" (in the years analyzed, which were 1960, 1962, 1964, and 1966). Nineteen schools ranked among the top twenty-five sources of medical students in each of those years. These nineteen schools, listed roughly in the order of their rank, are the following: Harvard, Michigan, Illinois, Columbia, Princeton, Cornell, Yale, Wisconsin, Dartmouth, Indi-ana, Texas, Pennsylvania University, California (Berke-ley), Minnesota, California (L.A.), Stanford, Ohio State, Emory, and Notre Dame. Assuming that these schools are the leading producers of top-quality medical students, the logic would appear to be inescapable that the major drive should be directed toward increasing black enrollment in the student bodies of these schools. It is indeed a promising trend that the black enrollment in these named colleges and universities is on the in-crease. There is no study to suggest, however, that the black student bodies at these particular colleges and universities are being specifically helped, encouraged, or motivated in the direction of medical or other scientific, technical career choices. But since these schools have represented the royal road of entry into American medical schools for white students, it would be a tragic oversight on the part of black student leadership, and college leadership at large, if black students did not travel the same route. This does not mean that a black premedical student would not receive very superior preparation for the study of medicine by attending one of the nation's many small but excellent colleges.

Black Medical Students

Table III (a reproduction of Table VII, Dove 1970) presents the black student enrollment in U.S. medical schools for selected years. One's attention is immediately drawn to the fact that from one year to the next, from 1968–1969 to 1969–1970, there was about a one-third increase in the number of black medical students, and that more than half of them were for the first time enrolled in predominantly white schools. Davis G. Johnson, Director of the AAMC Division of Student Affairs, discussed these statistics at the November 9, 1969, board meeting of National Medical Fellowships, Inc., held in Chicago, Illinois, and made the following additional comments: that while the overall increase of black enrollment went up more than a third of the total, the total freshman count rose from 266 to 440, or about twice the general rate of increase. Leaving out the students attending Howard and Meharry, the two predominantly Negro medical schools, the black medical student enrollment went from 292 to 546, or almost double from one year to the next; and limiting the count only to freshmen, there was almost a tripling from 124 to 320. Finally, while in 1968–1969 there had been thirty-one medical schools with no black freshmen, in 1969–1970 there were only twenty-one such schools. While there were thirty-six medical schools in 1968–1969 which had only one black medical student in any of the four years

TABLE III

Black Student Enrollment in
U.S. Medical Schools for Selected Years
1938–39 to 1969–70

Year	Total Enrollment	Number of Black Students	% Black Students	% of Total Black Enrollment in Predominantly White Schools
1938–1939	21,302	350	1.64	12.9
1947–1948	22,739	588	2.59	15.8
1948–1949	23,670	612	2.59	19.1
1949–1950	25,103	651	2.59	21.2
1950–1951	26,186	661	2.52	21.6
1951–1952	27,076	697	2.57	23.2
1952–1953	27,135	715	2.63	26.7
1955–1956	28,639	761	2.66	31.0
1968–1969	35,828	782	2.18	37.3
1969–1970	37,756	1,042	2.75	52.4

Source: 1. Dietrich C. Reitzes, *Negroes and Medicine*, Harvard University Press 1958

2. AAMC Fall 1969 Enrollment Questionnaire

of medical school, this was true only of eighteen of the hundred and one medical schools in 1969–1970. There was no school anywhere in the country with legal segregationist barriers preventing Negroes from attending, and even those schools with no blacks present stated that they would have accepted qualified applicants. If we go back only to 1955–1956, for purposes of comparison, for even at that time the legal barriers had come down, we can observe that thirty-two of the eighty-two medical schools in the country in that year were exclusively white (Reitzes 1958).[3]

By an ironic happenstance, only a few people who were well informed on medical educational affairs were aware of the important breakthrough from 1968–1969 to the 1969–1970 year in terms of the increased black enrollment. More attention was given the article by Crowley and Nicholson, "Negro Enrollment in Medical Schools"[4] *JAMA* 210:96, October 6, 1969. This report, prepared in behalf of the National Medical Association—American Medical Association Liaison Committee which had the charge of directing attention toward expanding opportunities for Negroes in the medical field, was made after a survey in the spring of 1969 of ninety-eight U.S. medical schools. The schools were asked to give the number of Negro students in each class, and to describe any special program aimed at increasing the number of black students in the school. Since at about that same time, the Association of American Medical Colleges had asked all the medical schools to write one-page summaries of any effort they were making along lines of recruitment, selection, special education, or special financial aid for minority group students (which appeared as a bulletin, *Minority Student Opportunities in United States Medical Schools 1969–1970*, June 1969),[5] Crowley and Nicholson used that study to supplement their own findings. Lacking the report of enrollment figures for 1969–1970, the

Crowley and Nicholson article was restrained in tone
and forecast, although they reported that schools were
increasing their black enrollments a little, " . . . from
1.95% in the class of 1968 to 2.87% in the 1972 class."
This increase trend is not so pronounced when the two
predominantly Negro schools are excluded. However,
there is a substantial increase in the percent of blacks
enrolled for the class of 1972. Forty percent of the total
black enrollment in medical schools (exclusive of
the predominantly Negro schools) is in the freshman
classes, suggesting there is "a positive result of increased recruiting efforts." The chief message, however,
was that there was cause for considerable concern that
only 2.39% of the 35,809 students in those ninety-eight
schools were Negro, that over three-fifths of them
(61.77%) were enrolled in the two predominantly
Negro medical schools, Howard with a black enrollment
of 73.82% and Meharry with 84.3%. And indeed there
is cause for concern that while one American in 560 becomes a doctor, among Negroes it is only one in 3,800.

Crowley and Nicholson went on to report that
eighty-four of the ninety-eight schools had at least one
black student in the 1968–1969 school year, and a total
of fifty-four schools had some form of special program
to recruit black students. Fifty of these schools already
had black students; another fourteen schools were planning to develop a new or expanded program (ten of
these already had black students), and twenty-nine had
no special program or plan to develop one at that
time (twenty-four of these had black students). In all,
twenty-six schools had programs aimed soundly, I believe, at strengthening the premedical academic preparation of black students. Of these, only nine schools
had the more special and, in my opinion, problematic
academic programs for these students after admission
to medical school. These programs included science
classes, summer laboratory workshops, summer research

assistantships, tutorial service, and a flexible curriculum allowing for individualized rates of progress. Of the fifty-four schools with programs in operation, only twenty-two provided special financial aid to the students. The public schools lagged behind the private schools in the recently stepped-up pace of recruiting activity and in the provision of financial aid. There was a note of pessimism, certainly warranted by the then available evidence, that the medical schools were still substantially segregated by "academic and economic circumstances" rather than by law or by administrative policy. It was also clear that the schools would have to provide a variety of academic assistance programs over the long range, reaching down to the high school level, as well as providing very much more specific financial assistance. This would be required in order not to penalize the potentially equal Negro applicant, decidedly disadvantaged in his home and family life and deprived of equal educational opportunity at earlier grade levels, all of which depress his scores on the Medical College Admissions Test and other such conventional test and learning measures.

There was considerable argument and controversy over how much weight should be given MCAT scores and grade-point averages of black applicants to medical schools, on whether these measures were or were not more valid indicators of present and future performance potential than the subjective impressions of several interviewers. In late 1969 and early 1970 there was still a great deal of feeling among organized black premedical and medical students that admissions policies and procedures were unfairly discriminatory, and a general feeling that practically no headway was being made. Surely the millennium had not come, but to minimize the achievement of a genuine opening-up of the schools to black admissions would be both unsound and wrong. There were those who felt that it was probably a fluke, a one-year occurrence which would not be sustained, and that not much should be made of it.

Two points required clarification. The lack of records on the number of Negro applicants, among the general pool of all applicants to medical schools, made it difficult to answer some rather simple questions. It was known, however, that over the past fifteen years or so, about half of all applicants to medical schools in the United States had been accepted into medical school (Dove 1970), since the applicant-acceptance ratio does not vary more than two-tenths of a percentage point from 1.9 during those years. It was estimated that there were six hundred black American applicants for the medical school classes which began in 1969, which means that if there was a total of four hundred and forty black freshmen in all medical schools in the fall of 1969, the black applicant acceptance was approximately 73% of all black applicants compared to about 50% for white applicants. This is the kind of statistic which is alluded to by those who believe that the medical school admissions committees are already lowering standards and unfairly favoring black applicants. This overlooks the obvious fact, however, that there was in 1968–1969 a total of 21,118 (minus six hundred black) applicants who were non-black. In other words, we come back again to familiar statistical territory: Only about 2.8% of all applicants to medical schools were black. The limitation of social, economic, political, and most of all, educational opportunity prevents Negroes from contributing more than about a fifth of their potential numbers to the nation's physician manpower team.

Why is it important to recruit black physicians? The shortage of black physicians, for one reason, is even more dramatic than the general physician shortage. Eleven percent of the population of the United States is black and this ought to represent at least their level of contribution to the top level of the health professions.

Moreover, it amounts to an institutionalization of inferiority that they should contribute many of their talented youth to the low-paid and low-status rungs of the health-career-field ladders, such as hospital aides, orderlies, etc. Further, blacks experience probably twice the statistically expected amount of most physical illness and suffering, and live in parts of most communities where physicians are in critically short supply. It is true, of course, that with the generalized easing of racially discriminatory barriers black physicians are no longer completely dependent on an underprivileged black clientele. A tenth of a nation is a very large human resource which no nation can afford to squander. This large body of potentially very able young people represents a major source of the physicians our country so desperately needs.

Why then, some may ask, do you not simply increase the size of the student body of the two predominantly black medical schools, and have them turn out two to three to four times as many black doctors as they do at present? The answer is as simple and as straightforward as the question. These schools do not possess the potential faculties, facilities, or budgets for such expansion; nor could they in the foreseeable future come up to par with the leading medical schools. The only genuine route to the production of several times the current number of highly qualified black physicians is to assure their preparation in the leading undergraduate colleges and medical schools, which for historical reasons have been more white than the common good requires. Moreover, it has not been generally known that the pattern of desegregation of medical schools has gradually crumbled during the past two decades. It did not really just begin in the past two years.

Both McLean and Reitzes remarked on this trend over ten years ago.[3] We can construct Table IV, utilizing their figures for the years up to 1956 and the recent

TABLE IV

Negro Medical Student Distribution

Year	Total Negro Students Enrolled	Negro Enrollment in White Schools	White Schools With Negro Students	Negro Percentage of all Medical Students
1947–1948	588	93	20	2.59
1955–1956	761	236	48	2.66
1969–1970	1,042	546	84	2.75

Source: Reitzes, Table 4, 1958; Dove, Table VII, 1970.

AAMC data for 1969–1970. Several trends are clear
from these figures in Table IV: Over the past twenty
years the number of Negro medical students enrolled
in medical schools has almost doubled, but the percentage of increase of Negro medical students to all medical
students has shown only a barely measurable increase,
and should probably be considered as having held at
essentially the same level. It is also clear that Howard
and Meharry have contributed relatively little to the
numerical doubling of black student enrollment during
the past twenty years. This doubling has come about
from the fact that white schools have increased their
total black enrollment about fivefold within the past
twenty years, and that four times as many different
white schools are now open that were formerly closed
to Negroes. Thus blacks were able to remain at a stand-
still of approximately two and a half percent of the medical student population, only because schools other than
Howard and Meharry began slowly to open up.

We have explored in the first chapter how Howard
and Meharry came into existence, but it is enough to
mention here that they came as a result of the refusal of
white schools to admit Negroes except on rare occa-
sions. They have produced black physicians where there
would have been none at all, but there has been a long
period of concern that the very existence of these
schools would constitute a barrier to desegregating the
system of medical education; that because they served
as a concession to racial segregation educationally and
socially, they would unwittingly become a force of re-
sistance to change.

The most complete presentation of the features of
Negro medical students was presented by Reitzes, who
had access to the most complete data available up to
that time. While these data are a little more than ten
years old, they present general trends which undoubtedly provide us with the best clues to a description of

the present group of Negro medical students. Howard University College of Medicine, and to an even greater extent Meharry Medical College, have traditionally accepted medical students with relatively inadequate preparation, who would probably not have been able to compete successfully at other schools. The better-prepared black students tended generally to attend the predominantly white medical schools, a trend going back a great many years. In Table V, we have a summary of data on the MCAT scores for all medical school applicants, accepted and rejected, as contrasted to scores for Negroes graduating from the two Negro schools, and Negroes graduating from the white schools.

These average figures indicate that by and large the graduates of Howard and Meharry, by conventional measures such as the Medical College Admissions Test, would not have been admitted to the average medical school, if we consider that their MCAT scores were lower than rejected applicants of other schools. Negro graduates from white medical schools scored higher than rejects from these schools, but scored below the average. Negro students in white medical schools who had also attended white undergraduate colleges scored still higher (Verbal 495, Quantitative 481, General Information 500, and Science 498), but still did not come up to the average for all medical students. The trend is unmistakable, however, that increased educational input yields increased output of learning and higher test scores. It is quite remarkable that this matter should have become so beclouded by value judgment, and have been seen in terms of race, which has in essence little or nothing to do with it. No better example could be found that the MCAT scores are at their basic core a measure of environmental learning opportunity than the fact that today the average scores of accepted medical school candidates at the very top schools are almost a hundred points higher than they were fifteen years ago.

TABLE V

Comparisons of MCAT Scores, 1950's Period

Test Section	All Applicants Accepted	All Applicants Rejected	Negro Graduates of Negro Schools	Negro Graduates from White Schools
Verbal	524	466	458	477
Quantitative	528	459	439	466
General Information	527	476	460	485
Science	522	454	454	484

A Modification from Reitzes Tables 21 and 38, (Reitzes 1958).

Admissions officers are frank in admitting that they are today rejecting white applicants in great numbers whom they would willingly have accepted, going by conventional learning and score measures alone, just a few years ago.

But this too gives us special cause for alarm, because the general quality of science teaching has increased markedly since Sputnik, both at high school and at college levels for the white student; but nothing of the kind has occurred in the schools attended by black high school and college students attending primarily black schools. The Macy Foundation[6] has done a very great deal here, indeed, through their support of the work of Cadbury's fifth post-baccalaureate year project, in which students from primarily black colleges would have a supplementary year of college on a more high-powered campus, in terms of science faculty and facilities and general faculty expertise. The Macy Foundation gave support also to the work of Severinghaus in strengthening premedical educational programs in the predominantly Negro colleges. The Macy Foundation sponsored a number of conferences, specifically designed to bring black premedical students and premedical advisors at black colleges into closer communication with the faculties of black and white medical colleges, and with black professionals in practice. This was done in order to bridge the obvious communication gaps which caused the inadequate utilization of developing opportunities.

One is forced to wonder if this was not a completely uphill fight. As Reitzes (1958) pointed out, the type of medical school the Negro student attends is definitely related to the type of undergraduate college he attends. Thus seventy percent of the students in Negro medical schools had their undergraduate training in Negro colleges, while only about thirty-two percent of Negro students from white medical schools had gone to Negro colleges. Also, while fifty-two percent of Negro premedical students from white colleges went to Negro medical schools, eighty-five percent of premedical students from Negro colleges went to Negro medical schools. Rather than attempting to upgrade the black schools and their programs, it would be more effective to open wider the doors of the predominantly white colleges both at undergraduate and medical school levels.

A somewhat futile effort has been made through the years to set up a separate network or pathway of black colleges, conceived to include an elite group, among the black schools sending students to medical schools. As Reitzes has pointed out, in 1954–55, fifty-one Negro colleges provided a total of four hundred and fifty-five applicants to medical schools, and ninety-five of all the acceptances. The top ten of these fifty-one schools, however, provided 62.4% of all applicants and 80% of all accepted applicants. Ranking the Negro colleges in terms of their total number of applicants and acceptances to all United States medical schools, we have the top twenty of the schools in the following order: Howard University, Lincoln University, Fisk University, Tennessee A. and M. State University, Morehouse College, Morgan State College, Hampton Institute, Virginia Union University, Virginia State College, Tougaloo College, Xavier University, West Virginia State College, North Carolina College at Durham, St. Augustine's College, Florida A. and M. University, Wiley College, Southern University, Alcorn A. and M. College, Clark College, and Central State College (Ohio). We find, however, that among well known schools that just missed inclusion are Dillard University, Wilberforce University, and Tuskegee Institute; and that a well-known school which supplied a number of high-quality Negro premedical students during the 1930's and 1940's, Talladega, is not among the first fifty Negro schools. The logic is inescapable that no great effort should be expended in trying to develop a strong network of elite black colleges just for black students who would then move on to the elite medical colleges of this country. The brave effort has already been made with no palpable result. Year by year, the most talented black students from the North or South are turning away from the segregated black colleges and attending integrated schools, a movement which is decidedly in their best interest.

During the late 1950's Reitzes noted that the five Negro colleges producing the greatest number of successful medical school applicants to all schools, as well as to Howard and Meharry, were the following, in rough order: Howard University, Lincoln University in Pennsylvania, Tennessee A. and M. State University, Morehouse College, and Hampton Institute. Over seventy-one percent of Meharry's applicants had attended Negro colleges, while only sixty-three percent of Howard's applicants were from Negro schools. Howard was at that time attracting a higher caliber of Negro premedical student, and among the ten colleges supplying the largest number of applicants were the College of the City of New York in third place, New York University in fifth place, and Detroit's Wayne State University in sixth place. Quite certainly there are fewer black applicants from such schools to Howard today, a matter we shall discuss at greater length later. It would appear inescapable that Howard and Meharry will become still more fully desegregated, welcoming white and black applicants equally rather than artificially holding down their acceptance of white applicants, a move which could only have the effect of moving those schools more fully into the mainstream of American medical education.

In the 1960's an important breakthrough occurred for American black males applying to medical schools. The National Medical Fellowships, Inc., which in the

1950's had primarily concerned itself with providing fellowships for Negroes, enabling them to take residency training and to become specialists, was awarded a Sloan Foundation grant to make awards to the ten best-qualified black applicants to medical schools nationwide. This grant was renewed each year for ten years, and Sloan Fellows were expected to have at least a B average and to have scored in the 500 range or better on the Medical College Admissions Test. It was the thought of the founder of NMF, the late Franklin C. McLean, that these students by their successful performance would open the doors of American medical schools to black students. These students performed well, and most of them had received their premedical preparation in the nation's strongest schools and were admitted to most of the leading medical schools in the country. Toward the end of the 1960's it was becoming clear from increasing numbers of applications for Sloan Fellowships, and with segregationist barriers almost down, that the time had come to mount a new program to provide financial aid not only to the select few, the very best, black premedical students but to all needy applicants who were able to be admitted to a medical school.

The policy statement of the AAMC in 1968 called on all medical schools to work toward the same ends: (1) to authorize immediate increases in the number of entering students; (2) to admit more students from groups and areas of the country not adequately represented; (3) to individualize the education of the physician, allowing for greater elective course work along multiple tracks or pathways during the four years, rather than the same set of required courses for all to complete in the same amount of time; (4) to permit the participation of students in the interdepartmental development of medical school curricula; and, (5) to assume responsibility for education and research in the organization and delivery of health care services.[7] It is clear that the presence of sizable representation of black and other minority group students in all medical schools could serve as a healthy catalyst to this kind of major improvement in design and function of undergraduate medical education.

The plan to expand the educational opportunities for greater numbers of blacks and other under-represented minority students took on more definite shape when a special AAMC Task Force issued its report on this subject in April 1970.[8] Despite the fact that 440 black freshmen entered all U.S. medical schools in the fall of 1969, a figure double the previous year's freshmen group, the basic relative shortage remained unchanged, since the total number (1,042) of all black medical students still made up only 2.75 percent of the total. It was anticipated that in the fall of 1970, 660 blacks would enter all medical schools, and this would bring the representation of minority group students up to 3.9 percent. It would require that by 1975 1,800 blacks and minority group students enroll as freshmen before these groups would comprise 11.9 percent, closer to their share of the population of the country as a whole. The chief barrier to that target was thought to be a financial one, since the overall amount of financial aid in scholarships and loans would have to be raised from five million dollars in 1970 to eighteen million in 1975. While it was believed important to recruit able students, to motivate them, and to retain them in the educational pathway leading to the M.D. degree, the provision of financial aid was seen as the primary problem.

Black Interns and Residents

Between 1947 and 1956 there was a marked improvement in postgraduate medical educational opportunity for the Negro medical school graduate (McLean's presentation in Reitzes, 1958). Just noting the graduates from Howard and Meharry alone, of whom there were

one hundred nineteen in 1947, forty-nine of them obtained internships in eight different white hospitals and
seventy served internships in various Negro hospitals,
only about a dozen of which had approved internship
training programs. Of the one hundred twenty-nine
Howard and Meharry graduates of 1956, seventy-seven
served internships in forty-six different white hospitals,
with only fifty-two men choosing internships in Negro
hospitals. By 1956, the shortage of residents was more
than twice as acute as the shortage of interns, and it became increasingly common for the Negro applicant to
have several choices of positions, none of which would
have been available only a few years before. It was becoming clear that our entire educational establishment,
while turning away half the students who applied to
medical schools, an unknown but presumably large
number of whom were really qualified, was simply fail-
ing to turn out anywhere near the number of doctors
necessary to run our nation's hospitals. We were not
only opening the doors of these hospitals to Negroes,
but the doors had already been opening for increased
numbers of graduates from foreign medical schools.

To illustrate, quoting from the *JAMA* Education
Number for 1969,[9] we note from the table on the com-
parative yearly status of internship and residency programs that in 1956 a total of 11,895 internships was offered, of which only 9,893 could be filled (1,988 being
filled by foreign graduates), but with 2,002 being left
vacant. A total of 28,528 residencies was offered, of
which only 23,012 were filled (4,753 of these being filled
by foreign graduates), leaving still 5,516 unfilled. By
1968–1969, of 14,112 internships offered only 10,464
were filled (3,270 of them by foreign graduates). Of
42,644 residencies offered 35,047 were filled (11,231 by
foreign graduates).

Just by observing the graph of the trend over the
twenty-year period from 1948–1968, we see plainly

that opportunities for residency training, even more than for internships, have either gone unfilled or have had to be filled by foreign graduates. Foreign medical graduates made up seventeen percent of the interns of medical-school-affiliated hospitals in 1968, a gain of three percent over the last year; and they comprised sixty-two percent of the interns at unaffiliated hospitals, a gain of twelve percent over the previous year. In all trainee positions foreign graduates were eighteen percent of all interns, sixty percent of all residents, and twenty-two percent of all "other trainees" in hospital programs in this country in 1968.

Of the 15,582 foreign graduate trainees in the United States in 1968, about a fifth were serving internships and the remaining four-fifths were residents. By country of origin and in rank-order for the first ten we have the following: Philippines (3,689 trainees), India (1,971), Korea (1,194), Thailand (721), Iran (659), Formosa (567), Spain (468), Argentina (431), Mexico (422), Germany (379). As Dorman[10] summarized this situation (1969), almost 7,000 graduates of foreign medical schools enter the U.S. each year (about 20% of of these are estimated, *JAMA* 1969 Education Number, to be U.S. or Canadian citizens who have studied abroad); about 1,400 foreign graduates become fully licensed to practice medicine; an unknown number of these graduates remain in the United States without licenses.

These developments had also the inevitable consequence of creating pressure for a merger between the fields of osteopathy and medicine.[11] Five schools of osteopathy in the United States graduate almost five hundred students a year, their students having come to them with less impressive credentials but with the same kind of premedical education. These students receive a variation of the usual medical school education which in recent decades has de-emphasized the role of the al-

leged musculoskeletal lesion. They are licensed to practice medicine and surgery in forty-two states; legisla-
tors, prominent laymen, and the general public accept
them practically on a par with M.D.'s, and they are coming to be almost the only general practitioners available
in those few states where they are most numerous.
Many of the osteopaths, having actually preferred to become physicians with an M.D. but not wanting to go
abroad to study, began to point out that the osteopathic
schools from which they graduated were probably better than some of the schools from which the foreign
medical graduates had come; that they further had an
advantage over the foreign graduate of "United States
cultural background, United States higher education,
and familiarity with medical English as spoken in the
United States." In 1962 the osteopaths in California
were given a chance to have their D.O. degrees transformed into M.D. degrees, and twenty-two hundred of
the twenty-four hundred became doctors of medicine
forthwith. The Los Angeles College of Osteopathic Physicians and Surgeons was converted in that same year
into a medical college, and in the State of California the
two professions merged into one. Resisted by some osteopaths as an attempt to take them over, increasingly
the American Medical Association and other organized
spokesmen are opening up opportunities for graduates
of osteopathic schools to serve internships and residencies in approved hospitals, and to join the medical
organizations, and convert their degrees. It is hard to
object to the view that the osteopathic physician's educational opportunities and facilities are inferior to those
available to the regular medical institutions, and that
the public interest is best served by improving their
educational opportunities rather than quibbling about
osteopaths' qualifications. Even so, a great number of
older and well established osteopaths, who are leaders
in their own power hierarchy, have all the traditional

reluctance of any leaders in relinquishing their apparent influence ("Congress on Medical Education, Osteopathy and Medicine," *JAMA* 209:85–96, July 7, 1969).[11]

Against this background one can understand the rather complete opening up of opportunity for Negroes to obtain internships and residency training opportunities. The *JAMA* Education Number for 1969 for the

TABLE VI

Negro U.S. Citizens Serving in Internship Programs

	Foreign Graduates Serving Internship	US or Canadian Graduates Serving Internship	Total
Alabama	2	. .	2
California	3	13	16
Colorado	. .	1	1
Connecticut	12	. .	12
District of Columbia	4	22	26
Florida	. .	1	1
Hawaii	. .	2	2
Illinois	6	5	11
Iowa	. .	1	1
Maryland	. .	1	1
Massachusetts	1	. .	1
Michigan	7	4	11
Missouri	. .	4	4
New York	8	35	43
Ohio	1	8	9
Oregon	. .	1	1
Pennsylvania	14	13	27
Puerto Rico	2	1	3
Rhode Island	14	. .	14
Texas	1	4	5
Utah	. .	1	1
Virginia	. .	1	1
Wisconsin	. .	1	1
Totals	75	119	194

JAMA, Nov. 24, 1969, Vol. 210, No. 8.

first time included tables showing the number and distribution of "Negro physicians who are United States citizens and who are interns and residents in U.S. hospitals." These Tables VI, VII, and VIII (reproductions of Tables 12, 13, and 14, *JAMA* 210:1550, November 24, 1969)[8] show that 801 Negro physicians, as of September 1968, were interns or residents. Of these, 563 or 70% graduated from U.S. or Canadian medical schools, and the remaining 238 or 30% graduated from foreign medical schools. It was a surprise, at least to me, to note that of the 194 interns, as many as 39% were graduates of foreign schools and only 61% were from U.S. or Canadian schools. Of the 607 residents, only 27% were graduates of foreign schools. All regions are represented, with the heavily populated urban areas better supplied, as might be expected. The rank-order of preference of residency seems not to be different from the ordinary choices: general surgery is first, followed by internal medicine, psychiatry, obstetrics-gynecology, and pathology. Of the total of 45,511 interns and residents on duty, the 801 Negroes comprised 1.8%; they represented 1.7% of the U.S. or Canadian graduates and 2.3% of foreign graduates serving as interns; they were 1.9% of U.S. or Canadian graduates who were residents and 1.5% of foreign graduate residents.

Since the best estimate (Dove 1970) is that 2.0% of those awarded the M.D. degree are Negro, and since the percentage of black medical students to all medical students within the past five years remains at the 2.0% level, this suggests that Negroes are not represented in the expected percentage; particularly in view of the fact that so large a component of reported interns and residents are from foreign medical schools. These figures, watched closely for the trend during the next few years, will show whether there is under-reporting. It is known that only about half as many Negro (9%) physicians as

TABLE VII

Negro U.S. Citizens Serving in Residency Programs by State

	Foreign Graduates Serving Residency	US or Canadian Graduates Serving Residency	Total
Alabama	15	2	17
Arizona	. .	2	2
California	1	67	68
Canal Zone	. .	1	1
Colorado	1	. .	1
Connecticut	3	2	5
Delaware	1	. .	1
District of Columbia	12	45	57
Florida	. .	3	3
Georgia	. .	2	2
Hawaii	. .	2	2
Illinois	6	27	33
Indiana	. .	3	3
Iowa	. .	3	3
Kansas	. .	3	3
Kentucky	. .	1	1
Louisiana	. .	3	3
Maine	5	. .	5
Maryland	3	14	17
Massachusetts	2	6	8
Michigan	14	25	39
Minnesota	. .	13	13
Missouri	. .	24	24
New Jersey	3	7	10
New York	24	90	114
North Carolina	3	3	6
Ohio	19	23	42
Oregon	. .	1	1
Pennsylvania	23	31	54
Puerto Rico	5	1	6
Rhode Island	5	2	7
Tennessee	14	1	15
Texas	1	28	29
Utah	. .	2	2
Vermont	. .	1	1
Virginia	3	. .	3

TABLE VII (Continued)

	Foreign Graduates Serving Residency	US or Canadian Graduates Serving Residency	Total
Washington	. .	2	2
Wisconsin	. .	4	4
Totals	163	444	607

JAMA, Nov. 24, 1969, Vol. 210, No. 8.

TABLE VIII

Negro U.S. Citizens Serving in Residency Programs, by Specialty

	Foreign Graduates Serving Residency	US or Canadian Graduates Serving Residency	Total
Anesthesiology	6	17	23
Child Psychiatry	. .	3	3
Dermatology	. .	10	10
General Practice	10	3	13
General Surgery	28	88	116
Internal Medicine	22	89	111
Neurological Surgery	2	4	6
Neurology	3	6	9
Obstetrics and Gynecology	14	51	65
Occupational Medicine	. .	4	4
Ophthalmology	1	15	16
Orthopedic Surgery	3	23	26
Otolaryngology	1	7	8
Pathology	23	13	36
Forensic Pathology	. .	8	8
Pediatrics	11	9	20
Physical Med. and Rehab.	4	3	7
Plastic Surgery	. .	1	1
Psychiatry	9	60	69
Radiology	7	13	20
Thoracic Surgery	4	2	6
Urology	2	7	9
Misc. or not Specified	13	8	21
Totals	163	444	607

JAMA, Nov. 24, 1969, Vol. 210, No. 8.

compared to all physicians (16%) are involved in approved internship or residency training,[13] despite the abundant opportunity.

Looking specifically at the field of psychiatry, and the opportunities there for residency training for Negroes, we are given an additional dimension on this problem. Negroes make up about 1% of all psychiatrists, but a recent census survey[12] of all residents showed that Negroes were 2% of all 3,284 psychiatry residents. This still is but a fraction of the opportunity available, as is shown by the following data on the ethnic or national origins of all psychiatric residents. It was found[12] that 78.8% were Caucasian, 7.9% were of Spanish extraction, 3.3% were East Indian, 3.7% Filipino, 2.5% Korean, 2% Negro, 1.1% Chinese, 0.2% Japanese, 3.5% other. There are those who would wonder whether whites and Negroes can understand each other well enough to be effective in the psychiatrist and patient relationship. These persons overlook the obvious fact that there are no basic or major cultural differences between black and white Americans. Such minor differences as there are do not in any way hamper professional relationships, as has been demonstrated amply. While exaggerated attention and emphasis has been given this matter of racial and cultural difference recently in this country, at the very same time, our psychiatric hospitals and training programs have been forced to turn to truly foreign countries and cultures in order to get their jobs done at all.

Black Physicians

In a statement in 1947 on *Medical Care and The Plight of the Negro*,[12] Montague Cobb pointed out that the accepted minimum standard of safety was one physician to 1,500 of population, and that the national average at that time was one to 750. He showed that the proportion of Negro physicians to Negro population in 1942 was one to 3,377, at a time when many white physicians preferred not to serve Negro patients, and the Negro medical man was very effectively confined to a nationally-dispersed professional ghetto. The national Negro population at that time was approximately 14 million, and there were approximately 4,000 Negro physicians. Comparing these figures with recent AAMC data (Dove 1970) relating to the year 1960, we note that on a nationwide basis there are 230,307 practicing physicians for a U.S. population of 201.2 million, which figures out roughly at about one physician to 1,500 of population. In other words, on a nationwide basis we have slipped considerably, while the estimated 5,038 practicing black physicians compared to 22.2 million black Americans figures out to one for every 3,700 of the black population, also a slip rather than a relative improvement in disparity of medical opportunity. Such comparisons are difficult to evaluate today, since the intervening decades have brought about considerable relaxation in color barriers affecting the behavior of blacks and whites both as professionals and as patients.

M. A. Haynes has written on the "Distribution of Black Physicians in the United States, 1967," utilizing as his primary source of data the 1968 Directory of the National Medical Association, the organization of black physicians which includes not only active but inactive members, as well as others.[14] This, while the best available source of data, probably leaves out a relatively greater number of black physicians who graduated from predominantly white medical schools, because more of them might have had little involvement in segregated medical communities. Nonetheless, he estimates that of an estimated 6,000 black physicians, 45.5% are Howard graduates, 37.9% are Meharry graduates, 15.1% are graduates of all other U.S. schools, 0.4% are graduates of Canadian medical schools, and 1.1% are foreign medical school graduates. In view of the fact that almost a third of the interns and residents were Negro U.S. citizens who had graduated from foreign medical schools (as shown by the data for 1968 cited in the *JAMA* Educational Number for 1969), one would be advised to be cautious in accepting the low figure Haynes cites of foreign medical school graduates.

As for the predominantly white medical schools with the greatest numbers of Negro graduates, they were ranked as follows: University of Illinois, University of Michigan, Wayne State University, Indiana University, Ohio State University, New York University, Harvard, Northwestern, Loma Linda University, and Chicago Medical School. California, New York, and the District of Columbia claimed the highest concentrations of black physicians. Howard graduates tended, in 17% of cases, to migrate to New York City to practice, or in the very same percentage, to remain in Washington, D.C. While 14% of Meharry graduates migrated to California, only 7% chose to remain in Tennessee where Meharry is located. Physicians continue to follow the migration patterns of the black population at large, a finding noted by P. B. Cornely in 1944,[15] which accounts for the fact that the black physician population of California has increased ninefold since 1942, as a reflection of the change in California's black population since that time. Similar trends are noticed in several states, dating from the 1940's.

Other interesting differences were noted between black physicians and physicians as a whole: Only 9% of black physicians are in training programs as contrasted to 16% for all physicians; only 2% of black physicians are in group practice as compared to 9.5% of all physicians; 61% of NMA members belong to the AMA as well (if we count the southern states which until very recently did not accept Negro members), compared to the finding that 69% of all physicians belong to the AMA. Thirty-nine percent of black physicians and 23% of all physicians are in general practice. The remainder limit their practice. This includes physicians who are certified by specialty boards, as well as those who are not. Among black physicians as a proportion of all physicians so specializing, we note by numerical rank-order: internal medicine 540 (1%), general surgery 479 (2%), obstetrics and gynecology 425 (2%), pediatrics 280 (2%), and radiology 109 (1%).

The much more dramatic figures relate to the number of men who have actually passed their specialty board certification examinations and become fully accredited specialists. Here we see a dramatic rise from 1947, at which time only ninety-three black physicians had passed specialty board examinations (Cobb 1947), to 1952, when 190 had passed these examinations; and 1957, when the number had risen sharply to 320 (McLean in Reitzes 1958), to a still more dramatic rise to 1,074 who had passed these examinations in 1967 (Haynes 1969). Haynes states that 31% of all physicians and 22% of black physicians are board-certified. If we but compare this with the fact that in 1947 Cobb observed that of approximately 4,000 black physicians, just under 100 were board-certified, this means that the rate of board certification for black physicians has risen almost tenfold, from about 2.5% to about 22% during the past twenty years. This is the strongest kind of evidence to support the contention that, given the postgraduate medical educational opportunity, blacks have made good use of them to upgrade their professional skills as they have moved to serve a more general public.

Summary

We began by discussing the long-term indications that the dual system of medical education which rigidly segregated whites from blacks is breaking down. We have noted that the black college enrollment generally is around six percent of the total, and that only forty percent of these students are now attending segregated all-black colleges. The predominantly white, elite colleges have traditionally supplied almost all successful applicants to the medical colleges of this country, and now that black college students are entering these schools, their chances for entering the mainstream of American medicine are much improved.

Almost eighty-five percent of all black medical students had until recently attended Howard or Meharry, the two predominantly black medical schools; but just within the past year or two the trend has been reversed, so that now just over half of all the black medical students are attending racially integrated, predominantly white, medical schools. Analysis shows that over the past few decades Howard and Meharry did not take substantially greater numbers of black students because of limitations in faculty, facilities, budgets, and other resources. The percentage of black medical students to the whole was maintained at approximately 2.5%, only by the fact that the predominantly white schools took in four times as many students, and that four times as many predominantly white schools opened their doors to black applicants. (See Table IV, figures on Negro Enrollment in White Schools.)

The severe shortage of interns and residents not only led to large numbers of vacancies in these positions, but to increasingly large numbers of graduates from foreign medical schools who have become absolutely necessary to the operation of our hospitals. The shortage has also stimulated movements toward the merger of osteopaths with regular physicians, with many actual and proposed schemes to allow osteopaths to be automatically declared doctors of medicine and to welcome them into internships, residencies, and staff positions previously open only to regular physicians. While only twenty years ago it would have been difficult for Negro medical school graduates to find internships or residences except in two dozen approved settings, half of them segregated, the overwhelming number of black medical school graduates have for some time had their postgraduate training in racially integrated hospital settings. There is still indication, however, that Negro graduates are not fully involved in the expected numbers or proportions in these postgraduate positions.

There is also an indication that the number of U.S. Negro citizens who pursue their medical education abroad may have been dramatically underestimated, since we are only now beginning to collect statistical data on the professional involvement of blacks.

In view of the steadily decreasing racial barriers that up to now have limited freedom of movement of blacks and whites who would be able to use each other in physician-patient relationships, Negroes still are under-represented in the medical profession in terms of their proportion of the general population, relative interest in pursuing medical careers, relative need for medical services, and relative demand for the black physicians' services.

There have been marked movements toward increasing professional competence, as judged by dramatic increases in proportions of black physicians who specialize in the various medical specialties, almost up to a level of their total representation within the general pool of physicians within the past two decades.

Further representation of Negroes among the physician manpower of the country can be expected to come from a continuation of the process which is already under way, the complete removal of all segregationist policies from all American medical schools, hospitals and other training institutions, and from the colleges where the best premedical preparation can be obtained.

III

Producing Qualified Black
Applicants from High School

Introduction

Fifteen years ago, Richard L. Plaut, then President of the National Scholarship Service and Fund for Negro Students, was convinced that if all racial discriminatory barriers to college enrollment for Negroes were removed overnight, and if all their financial needs were met at the same time, there would not ensue any significant increase in the number of Negroes entering the nation's first-class colleges, graduate or professional schools. The primary reason: too few Negroes were graduating from academic high schools with the standard academic curriculum preparation for college and preprofessional work, and with grade-point averages and college board scores at a minimal level acceptable to the best schools. Established in 1948 for the specific purpose of increasing the enrollment of Negroes in interracial colleges, and having made contact with most of the leading colleges in the country to determine what they would provide and expect of the student, NSSFNS had placed about twelve thousand students within seventeen years in a total of four hundred and fifty of the nation's colleges. The colleges were willing to accept high school graduates whose credentials were not quite up to those of their average applicant, the colleges agreeing that this was a reflection of cultural lacks in the student's past life and family experience, as well as a reflection of poor education received in segregated ghetto neighborhoods. But NSSFNS made every effort to place only those students who came close to acceptance standards. NSSFNS usually was not able to place more than a fifth of the students who would have been offered college acceptances, preferring not to refer to colleges those applicants who would have little chance of competing successfully with other students. The NSSFNS program was a success by all measures. Their nine percent college drop-out rate compared with a national average of forty percent and when they graduated, the NSSFNS students were on an academic par with their classmates or were above average.[1]

The problem, as Plaut saw it, was to go down into the earlier grades of high school; to identify bright students from this much larger pool; to increase the number of survivors at the twelfth year by giving younger students the special counseling, intellectual enrichment, and other support they required. His agency joined several others in actually demonstrating that in a substandard junior high school—completely segregated and in Harlem—a program of intensified support and enrichment was able several years later to cut the drop-out rate in half and to double the number of youngsters enrolling in college. This served as a model for the scholarship program conducted by the Provident Clinical Society of Brooklyn, led by its Scholarship Committee of which the author was chairman, with a group of youngsters in Bedford-Stuyvesant from 1963 through 1969.

The Provident Clinical Society of Brooklyn, made up of physicians, dentists, and pharmacists, and almost one hundred percent Negro, is one of the local branches of the National Medical Association. It has been in existence, except for a few years of organizational disruption, for almost fifty years. Having been a member of this organization myself for over twenty years, I can state that it has tried with success not to be primarily social, but rather to devote itself to the health needs of the Negro community as well as to special problems of Negro practitioners. Most of us reacted without surprise to the news that only 500, or about 2.6%, of New York City's 19,000 physicians were Negro in 1963, representing a smaller absolute number than ten years earlier. Moreover, only 70 Negro physicians that year had hospital staff appointments or privileges at an approved hospital.[2]

Negro representation in the various professions in New York City have followed certain trends, as reported in the 1966 edition of *The Negro Handbook*.[3] The Negro population of New York City in 1960 was roughly 14% of the total; Negroes had been 3% of all professional workers in the city in 1950 and this had risen to 5% in 1960, most of the increase being accounted for by increased numbers of social workers and of nurses. There was a drop by one-fourth in the number of Negro clergymen, from 671 to 496, in the decade from 1950 to 1960. Negroes generally showed great numerical increases in professions which traditionally attract women—social work (22%), nursing (17%), and teaching—but large numbers of Negro men also entered these fields. In 1960 the number of Negro male social workers and teachers exceeded the total number of all other Negro male professionals combined. Negroes were less than 6% of all the following fields: dentists, librarians, physicians natural scientists, and teachers. They were less than 2% of all accountants, college faculty members, engineers, lawyers, and pharmacists.

Provident's Scholarship Program

In 1963, not only in Brooklyn but elsewhere, feeling was strong that there should be no further delay in granting full civil rights to Negroes, and that there was no way to separate the struggle for health rights from educational rights, or the rights to dignified jobs and homes. The Provident Clinical Society found itself supporting a variety of actions: to picket the construction site at the State University of New York's Downstate Medical Center's new hospital, for example, in order to bring pressure on the construction unions to allow Negroes into their apprenticeship training programs; to support the boycott of public schools urging the Board of Education to mount a feasible plan for desegregating the schools and providing quality education; to support voter-registration proposals and campaigns. We were also particularly concerned, in Provident, to note that although half a dozen of us were faculty members at Downstate, there had not been a Negro in the freshman class of the medical school for three years. Moreover, it seemed true that no qualified applicant had presented himself or herself. With this problem in mind, the Provident Clinical Society decided in the fall of 1963 to begin a program for the early identification and support of able junior high school students who might choose a medical or other health career.

The aim was that our 36-member volunteers would function as Big Brothers in providing supportive friendship to a similar number of students by seeing them regularly in our offices or homes, or in the student's home, showing interest in the student's work, and helping either directly by tutoring or by arranging for the necessary help. Also we were to refer the student or members of his family for necessary health or social services which might be required during times of family crisis. For problems requiring special services, we made arrangements for the Bedford Mental Health Clinic to accept referrals of situations needing social casework or brief psychotherapy. In addition, the Bedford Mental Health Clinic social workers maintained regular contact with the youngsters' school guidance counselors, after each marking period, in order to know the earliest signs of difficulty. After the first year we had the additional services of a group worker from the Christian Herald Youth Services Program, through which many of the students received summer camp experiences. The group worker maintained contact with these students in a year-around program of activity. A number of other agencies provided summer camp placement, or other concrete services for our group. The main provision, however, was to be the one-to-one relationship between the student and his sponsor (there were twenty-nine boys who had men-sponsors, and seven girls who had women-sponsors). Each sponsor also agreed to contribute $1,000 personally to a scholarship fund, understanding that this amount would go to each student who graduated from high school and was enrolled into college.[4] Looking over the record of the six years from 1963 to 1969 when the youngsters graduated from high school, and appraising the amount of supportive relationship the various sponsors contributed to their students, we can conclude that about one-fourth of the sponsors extended considerable effort on behalf of their students; another quarter did very little; and the remainder was between those extremes.

How were the youngsters picked? We asked and promptly received the interest and support of the assistant superintendent of schools in one of the Bedford-Stuyvesant school districts. We held a conference with the seventh-grade guidance counselors in each of the seven junior high schools of that school district. We were interested in working with youngsters who were high-average, or preferably superior, in ability by conventional intelligence test scores or learning achievement tests, feeling that this would be a minimal index of their ability. In at least half the instances we wanted students who were working well and steadily earning good grades. We included only those who had no immediate family relative who had ever gone to college, because we wanted to help those in greatest need.

The counselors interviewed approximately two hundred youngsters and parents before selecting the thirty-six youngsters who most completely met our description of situations in which we thought we would be most helpful. We did not set as a requirement that the youngsters should have a definite interest in medicine, dentistry, pharmacy, nursing, or any health career; because we knew that at the seventh-grade level this would be premature as well as unsound. There was strong feeling among many in Provident that we should pick at least some students who were not performing well, despite indications of talent (and at least a quarter of them were from families receiving public assistance), to be sure that we were intervening with a group of youngsters who would not be likely to survive without our intervention. We knew that the high school dropout rate from ghetto high schools was over fifty percent for initial seventh graders. We were limited in the number of students selected by the number of sponsors who volunteered. The schools assured us that at least one hundred of the youngsters interviewed would have been suitable for inclusion.

The schools continued to maintain active interest and concern, especially as the students progressed from the seventh through the eighth and ninth grades, because they usually remained within the same school jurisdiction. However, starting with a few students who went into high schools from the eighth grade, and with the remainder who entered high schools after the ninth grade, it became almost impossible to maintain effective communication with guidance counselors in all the various high schools in which our students were enrolled. Furthermore, for almost all our students it was their first experience attending a school outside their ghetto neighborhood, and they began to encounter stiffer academic competition. Throughout the tenth, eleventh, and twelfth years many of our students came close to dropping the academic curriculum. We provided several programs of special remedial work in English and in mathematics throughout the high school years, all voluntary, but with considerable effort to persuade students who needed it most to use the service. It was rather clear that the quarter of our students who were from the beginning very able remained that way; only one or two previously mediocre or poor students became consistently good students; while by and large the quarter of the students who were poor scholars with poor work habits remained so throughout.

As we surveyed our efforts in the fall of 1969, there seemed to be no doubt that our intervention had been a success. Of our thirty-six students, thirty-two had graduated from high school. Of the thirty-two high school graduates, twenty-nine were enrolled in college. We knew that another four students might be helped to enter college by our continued effort. This excellent start did not give us any great yield for medicine or the health field, as one might have anticipated. At the time they graduated from high school, only four or five students had definite interests in medicine, while ten to a dozen had specific interests in engineering, with the remainder uncertain. All but one who will enter law, and another who will enter the ministry, were primarily interested in some scientific field. With the next few years, an unknown number of these students may shift into health or allied medical fields, or they will at least retain the potential of doing so at some later time if they should so choose. The members of Provident were proud of their accomplishment at any rate, for it seemed remarkable that eight-ninths of our youngsters had graduated from high school and seven-ninths were enrolled in college, as a result of our efforts and special efforts of others we could rally in their behalf. During their senior year the National Scholarship Service and Fund for Negro Students had arranged for one of their staff to interview each student to help the student make his choice of college. All but two students picked an inter-racial college.

The anticipated shift in career interest did in fact occur during their first year of college work. Most students became aware of the fact that engineering, which sounded glamorous to them as high school students, did not really hold a great deal of promise in terms of attractive and well-paid jobs with opportunities for advancement and financial security. Without question the students were beginning to hear the news of increased opportunities for blacks in medicine, and the fact of their previous association with those of us in the Provident Clinical Society served to give this greater meaning for them. Whereas the year before only four or five of them had expressed interest in medical careers, ten of them expressed such interest by the summer of 1970. In fact, six of the Provident students had summer jobs during the summer of 1970 at the Cornell University Medical Center in order to have an experience upon which to base their further career choices.

Evaluating the Effect of the Program

Several years of partnership in working on the Provident Scholarship Program had led to a close feeling of teamwork between members of the Scholarship Committee, myself, and Dr. Abraham Tauchner, Assistant Superintendent of the 16th School District, and his main staff. As we discussed various ways of evaluating the effectiveness of our intervention in supporting the educational careers of the thirty-six students, it became necessary for members of Dr. Tauchner's staff to conduct an additional study, which was effectively undertaken by Marie O'Connell with the assistance of Sidney

Rosen.[5] The decision was made to compare our thirty-six Provident youngsters with all youngsters who were in the brightest section of the seventh grade in the same year (1963) they were first selected. All of this contrast group were initially high in both test ability and in scholarship performance, and were from three of the seven schools from which our youngsters were drawn. We wanted to see how many of these high-ability and high-performance youngsters from some of the same schools went on to graduate and to enter college six years later. It will be recalled that of our Provident youngsters, only about a quarter showed high ability and were high performers, the rest of our group being of high ability, but with average or even low performance.

One of the three junior high schools selected for the contrast was on the edge of Bedford-Stuyvesant, which meant that in the case of that particular school, from seventy-five to eighty percent of all the student body was made up of lower-middle-class, stable, Italian and German families, with only twenty to twenty-five percent Negro students. In 1963–1964, there had been thirty-four students enrolled in their 7–1 (or best) group. Of this number only two students transferred to another junior high school during the seventh, eighth, or ninth grades. Of the thirty-four, twenty-eight went on to senior high school; eighteen were known to have graduated from high school (ten with the academic diploma), and eleven had applied to college. The Board of Education does not ordinarily keep records of whether or not students applying for college admission are actually accepted, or where. Junior high schools ordinarily have no way of checking on what happens to students once they go on to senior high school. It became extremely difficult to trace students who transferred from one senior high school to another within the city, and practically impossible to trace students who left the city. Therefore we have no way of knowing exactly what happened to the ten students who went into senior high school but did not graduate, although there were indications that two of these may have been drop-outs, with the remainder representing cases too difficult to trace. In other words, we have in this, the most stable and racially integrated of the three contrast schools, an indication that, of their best 1963 seventh graders, only eighteen out of thirty-four were high school graduates, and it seemed that only eleven had applied to colleges.

The next junior high school was in the middle of Bedford-Stuyvesant and was made up of ninety-seven percent Negro, two percent Puerto Rican, and one percent other enrollment. Their brightest 7–1 group consisted of forty-one students. There had been considerable residential mobility, with twelve different students transferring at least once to another junior high school during the seventh, eighth, or ninth grades. Of the forty-one, thirty-four went on to senior high school; but only twelve were known to have graduated (only four with the academic diploma), and only seven in all had applied to college. Not a third of them had graduated from high school, compared to half the students from the more stable junior high; only a sixth applied to college, compared to a third from the more stable junior high school.

This impression was confirmed by looking at the third junior high school, made up of eighty percent Negro and twenty percent Puerto Rican enrollment. Their 1963 class for 7–1 students contained thirty-eight students. Again there was considerable residential mobility, with eleven children moving to at least one other junior high school during grades seven, eight, or nine. Of the thirty-eight, thirty-one went on to senior high school; twelve were known to have graduated (ten with academic diplomas), and ten had applied to college. The figures are just a very slight amount better than those of the junior high school just previously mentioned.

Taken altogether, there were one hundred thirty-three youngsters in grade 7–1 in 1963–1964 in the three junior high schools reviewed; ninety-three were known to have gone to senior high school; only forty-three were known to have graduated from high school in June 1969; only twenty-eight are known to have applied to college. Far fewer than half graduated from high school; only a quarter applied to college, and we can be certain that not all of these were actually enrolled into college. These findings carried us beyond considerations on the particular Provident study to the possibility of the need for major improvement in planning several of the large and costly programs of compensatory intervention for children attending schools in ghetto neighborhoods.

Demonstrated Achievement Versus Demonstrated Need

It was apparent from the foregoing comparison, not only that our intervention with the thirty-six Provident Program students had been effective, but that our efforts might have been more effective still, had we confined ourselves to straightforward high-achieving youngsters in the 7–1 classes, who would have elected to be in the program. Most educational programs for Negroes have had to grapple with the question of whether or not to aim for quality or quantity of candidates for higher education. Sometimes there is no necessity for making such a forced choice at all, but only seldom do we have a chance to examine the consequences of such decisions.

One would not have anticipated that a group of very able and very high-performing seventh graders, at age thirteen, would suffer a fifty-fifty chance of losing their academic achievement orientation and performance abilities by the time they would be expected to graduate from high school. Indeed, the more general presumption in the minds of most people would be that any student doing well as a seventh grader will have no need for any special program because the youngster himself, his family, and the school system all seem to be lined up supportively with each other. Why were they thrown off balance and out of line in such great frequency? Possible answers are: They are not provided with enough significant individualized or cultural support in depth to protect them from adverse environmental and group norms, for this seems to have been the main provision we made for our Provident students; and they may have been unable to stand up competitively with youngsters who had been provided with superior schooling in better neighborhood schools for greater periods in earlier years. Whatever the reasons, the fact remains that public educational policy and public funds, at least in New York City, are probably not being spent to assure the greatest likelihood of return.

H. H. Davidson's and J. W. Greenberg's "Traits of School Achievers From a Deprived Background", one of the few studies of the subject,[6] was an attempt to focus attention on certain facts. While it is well known that children from low-income families do less well academically than children from middle- and high-income families, it is less well known that some children from low-income families are high academic achievers. Moreover, some of these are Negro. Davidson and Greenberg selected eighty of these high-achieving youngsters, fifth graders from Central Harlem schools, and studied them in comparison with eighty low achievers from similar schools. The high achievers were, on average, reading one-and-a-half years above grade; while the low achievers were about two years below grade, with slightly less separation between the two groups in arithmetic. The two groups of youngsters were given an extensive battery of psychological tests. In addition, teacher evaluations of achievement behavior had to match the test scores. The youngsters were interviewed; visits were made to the home and parents were interviewed; and there were physical examinations and medical histories taken by pediatricians.

There were several important findings: the high and low achievers could not be separated on the basis of attitude or motivation demonstrated, since both groups expressed great interest in learning. Successful achievement for low-income youngsters is apparently associated with the same personality variables that distinguish high from low achievement in the middle-income class. High achievers tend to have better verbal skills, to have a good self concept, adequate controls, directed effort, acceptance of reasonable authority demands, better school attendance records, more parental concern for education, more anxiety about performing well. Generally their coping mechanisms are more effective, although at times they are too controlled and too conforming. While it is possible, the authors conclude, that the high achievers started out with an initial advantage over the low achievers, it is even more likely that the school system's practice of homogeneous ability grouping, accompanied by the general tendency on the part of teachers to give greater approval to the children rated as brighter, tends to exaggerate the initial difference.

The New York City public school system does not have any special program or effort to maintain high levels of achievement among ghetto children identified as high achievers at elementary school grades. They are not systematically followed into the junior high school years, and into the senior high schools, to the point of college admission. In fact, even for the youngster who is exceptionally bright and placed in a class for the intellectually gifted in elementary school, or into one of the so-called Special Program Classes for gifted children in the junior high school years, there is no special guidance. Even these youngsters may end up attending a vocational school, or may end up with a general diploma, without having taken courses to prepare him for college application, and without special discussions about college with his parents.

While these youngsters are being overlooked, we find that large amounts of money and staff effort are spent to work with youngsters identified not so much because they have clearly demonstrated scholarship ability, but because they have clearly demonstrated financial need. To illustrate, the College Bound program for the New York City schools aims to increase the flow of low-income, minority-group students into college. Several thousand students from the tenth, eleventh, and twelfth grades are in that program, which is set up to provide a range of small classes, remedial tutoring, family counseling, and individual supports. In order to enter the program there must be the subjective impression of several teachers that the youngster has college-level potential ability, but the youngster must be at least two years behind in reading and arithmetic computational skills, and must come from a family which is at or below the poverty line.

From a review of the *1970–71 Upward Bound Guidelines* from the U.S. Department of Health, Education, and Welfare's Office of Education (1969)[7] such students must in ninety percent of the instances come from such families as, let us say, a nonfarm family of four earning no more than $3,600, or a farm family earning $3,000 or less. Only ten percent of the students may come from nonfarm families with earnings as great as $4,700 and in farm families this can go to $3,500. The guidelines go on to inform us that these students should all be considered as "academic risks" for college education, to such an extent that their high school records would not have warranted acceptance into either a two-year or a four-year college without the Upward Bound program. The student is "a young person with academic potential constrained by his poverty background, and one for whom conventional education has had little relevance. The student is likely to be apathetic or even hostile to education—unable to release his real talent. He is likely to have shunned academic achievement or even adequacy because he has not participated meaningfully in an educational experience. Generally, the potential that the student possesses does not show in traditional educational measurements, such as standardized test scores or grades, but may be discovered more readily through the intuitive judgments of those people who know him. . . ." It is a fact that after several years of inclusion in these programs, some of these students are learning and achieving on or above grade. Working with the so-called "high-risk" student has, however, become such a fad, that students who are not special risks receive a low priority, or none at all, in the minds of many who are in charge of planning or financing these special services.

It should not be surprising to note that in California a deliberate policy was pursued, at least at one college, to select for college admission those minority-group youngsters who had records of being drop-outs, who had police records, and who had been students with "C" averages or below, and who professed no interest in college in their first interview.[8] It should not require extended comment for me to point out that such students would be unsuitable candidates for the medical profession.

The Need for New Guidelines in Compensatory Education Programs

All of this would be understandable and even laudatory if there were no black students in the public school system who are able, achieving, performing, and conventionally capable of competing with any other students anywhere. Such students are identifiable, exist in great numbers, but are being passed over for other students who are of demonstrable high risk, as a condition for their acceptance. It sounds absolutely as though it were a scheme to deprive the urban blacks of the trained leadership of their most able people. And yet this kind of program would be supported by a number of loudly vocal "black leaders" who insist on special educational programs suitable only for black youngsters, although many of these suggestions must originate with whites who promote separatist philosophies.

Responsible Negro leaders and scholars are almost unanimous in opposing this special separatist upsurge, but the point of view of a conspicuous few has gained considerable popularity. In a recent interview reported in the *Wall Street Journal,* Kenneth Clark, the Negro psychologist, was asked if he thought the educational needs of whites, blacks, Indians, or Mexican-Americans were significantly different. He replied in the negative and added that the effective compensatory programs with which he was familiar were nothing more than programs in which children were being well taught by accepted methods. He was also asked, because there has been a strident assertion by a very few in this regard, whether he favored teaching black dialect in the schools and the attempt to give Negro dialect the status of a foreign language, to which he said, "I do not believe that you can make the deviations and the variants the standards."[9] Here again, not only would most educated Negroes agree with Clark, but they would be horrified at the prospect that in the name of black pride their youngsters were being routinely taught a substandard form of English under the pretense that it represented their very own language.

Much of the discussion on compensatory programs

for black children in ghetto neighborhood schools has been conducted at the unbelievably low level of whether there was a need for special programs for the children and their families, or whether there was a need for a change in the way the school system operates in its efforts to teach. Obviously there is a need for both kinds of change. Equally clear is the fact that compensatory programs directed toward the child should begin as early in the child's life as possible, that a public education program worthy of its name should continue throughout the adult life span until death, there being no logical point at which one should experience no further need for learning. Within those general outlines, it would also follow that programs of instruction at high school levels could be made more rigorous if the children were subjected to a uniform high standard of schooling during the elementary school years. Similarly, rigorous schooling in the high school years would preclude the need for elaborate remedial tutorial programs at the college level. Most of all, there is a realistic need to face the fact that children, black or white, cannot learn what they have not been taught. The chief differences which have separated black and white youngsters in terms of learning achievement have rested on the solid base of their differential access to an environment of teachers, formally or informally designated or not mentioned as such.

But the most glaring fact of all is that those minority group, low-income children who are high achievers, who have comfortably accepted and introjected, middle-income family life styles with respect to learning and work habits, are treated as if they do not exist. They are simply ignored. And yet in one Brooklyn school district alone, District 16 with which I am most intimately acquainted, in the fall of 1969 there were no fewer than nine hundred and fifty intellectually gifted children in grades one through nine, with almost nothing in the way of a special program of support for them or their families to guide and maximize their subsequent school and college career. This does not include the additional several thousand students who were in the brightest tracks of their various school grades. This is to say, the system of tracking students in the public school system of New York may be criticized with justification on a number of grounds. In the opinion of some, it produces the very superiority it claims to measure and reward. Moreover, in the case of ghetto children, even after the youngsters are put into the higher level tracks or group-ings, there is no follow-up or payoff. The brighter ones are as lost and unheard of as the so-called duller ones.

Open admission to the New York City college sys-tem—the notion that just any student at all who applies should be admitted and possibly graduated—does not make a favorable impression as a plausible or desirable policy. However, the one group of students for whom such a system would work best are the very ones I have just described above, those students in the brightest tracks of the elementary and junior high grades. Rather than that, only about a fifth to a quarter of these stu-dents in any given year choose to take the special ex-aminations required to gain entrance into the city's elite high schools from which college admission is practically assured—Brooklyn Technical High School, Bronx High School of Science, Stuyvesant, and Hunter College. The schools are entirely passive in this, leaving the initiative to the child and his family to request these examina-tions. Still other counselors are afraid their students will do poorly there against tough competition. These chil-dren are for the most part scheduled to attend high schools determined by their address, without paying at-tention to the strengths or weaknesses or reputation of that high school's teaching program. If the youngster rejects that school assignment, there is no means of fol-lowing it up with the child or his family or his high school, that he should take the academic curriculum rather than one of the non-college-oriented curricula. Clearly there should be early identification of able youngsters and straight-through planning and curriculum guidance throughout the school years, pointing those talented ones to assured college entrance to a four-year college. Less able students could be moved toward two-year colleges, with an opportunity to move to a four-year college if their work improves; while for other students college would not be the appropriate plan.

As the nation learned from the Coleman Report of 1966, the average Negro twelfth-grade student in the northeastern part of the country, the most favored, is reading at a ninth-grade level and is doing mathematics at the seventh-grade level. This is a result of denial of equality of educational opportunity, for the learning achievement gap separating urban Negroes in the Northeast from Negroes in the rural South is as great as the gap between urban Negroes and whites. As Coleman has discussed the matter further,[10] when public education began to appear in Europe and the United States in the early nineteenth century, there was no uniform idea of what equality of educational opportunity was to be. In England the system was designed to provide differentiated educational opportunity appropriate to one's station in life, and this is the meaning it took in this country so far as Negroes were concerned. Only since the 1954 Supreme Court decisions against segregated schools can it be said that the educational establishment is being compelled to assume responsibility for the gaps in learning achievements of deprived youngsters, and to take steps to educate all children effectively The factors affecting the learning achievement of black students are the same, and are in the same order of importance as those affecting white students:

facilities and curriculum least, teacher-quality next, and backgrounds of fellow students most.

It would follow from the above analysis that many of the supported policies to improve ghetto education may be of less relevance than commonly supposed; for example, placing the schools under local neighborhood control, or having all black principals and teachers, even if there were enough to go around. It is unlikely that these measures, taken alone, could promote significantly greater amounts of learning achievement. But to return again to the earlier finding, there should be a plan to identify those students who are high achievers as early as possible, to arrange for their orderly transfer into the strongest possible schools in whatever neighborhoods those schools are located. This we must do if we are to be guided by the best knowledge currently at hand.

Summary

Programs to stimulate and increase the enrollment of Negroes in the top colleges at undergraduate, graduate, and professional school level all depend on increasing the number of Negro graduates from strong academic high schools.

Several demonstrations have shown, including the one reported here with thirty-six junior high school students from Bedford-Stuyvesant, that long-term, individualized, supportive guidance and friendship can very significantly increase the likelihood that bright Negro youngsters will graduate from high school and go on to college.

Many compensatory education programs for ghetto youth are poorly planned because they are designed to reach only youngsters from the most impoverished families, who have already suffered serious learning disabilities, and who have weak or uncertain motivations for higher education.

Large numbers of children from minority group, low-income families are high in learning achievement and in conventionally measured intelligence, but these youngsters have few programs set up to further their entry into colleges. They represent a major untapped resource for the nation's medical manpower needs.

IV

Work with Black Premedical Students

The Cornell-Hampton Collaboration

During 1968, with increased attention to the need for active programs of recruitment for black students in most of the leading medical schools, Cornell University began to move in that direction. The Executive Faculty, the chief governing body for the medical school, appointed a faculty committee[1] to explore the development of such a program. Simultaneously and independently at first, an active committee[2] of medical students was also working on a proposal for "Disadvantaged Students." These two committees of faculty and of students very soon began to work together to come to the set of final recommendations which were approved by the Executive Faculty in November of 1968. In essence it was agreed that: (1) A program should go into operation during 1969–1970 and should aim at the active recruitment of more than token numbers of black students to the medical school; approximately one-tenth of each class would be considered a realistic goal. (2) The director of such a program should be a full-time person with experience in medicine, medical education, counseling, and administration; he would be a member of the Dean's staff and preferably hold a faculty appointment as well. (3) A supplementary program should be devised, preferably with black premedical students prior to their coming to medical school to avoid their being treated as a "special" group. (4) Their full financial needs would be met, in order to remove this obvious barrier to their academic success.[3]

An outgrowth of these recommendations was my decision to come to Cornell in June 1969, as Assistant Dean of the Medical College (a year later I was promoted to Associate Dean), and as Associate Professor of Psychiatry. A second outcome was the decision to conduct a special program of ten-week summer research fellowships for black premedical students who had just completed their junior year. Such students would normally be about to decide to what schools they should apply, would have a remaining year of premedical work to remedy any weakness in their preparation, and would have a preview experience of what it might be like to be a black student at the Cornell Medical Center. Dean John Deitrick, then Dean of the Medical School, and Dr. Jerome Holland, then President of Hampton Institute and a Trustee of Cornell University, agreed that their two schools would collaborate in this special program. Ten Hampton post-junior premedical students were to be engaged in a variety of research activities, with individual medical school faculty members from different departments as sponsors. This was a natural development, inasmuch as similar summer fellowships are ordinarily held by a number of Cornell's medical students and predoctoral students from the Graduate School of Medical Sciences. The Hampton students were housed in the regular medical students' dormitory, and they received a $100-per-week stipend to defray living costs and provide a small amount of savings.

A series of seminars, scheduled twice weekly with the author as leader, provided information on medical careers and included such topics as procedure for application to medical schools and how to obtain financial aid. It was especially arranged that black physicians in the various specialties, working in the metropolitan area, were included among the professionals outlining medical career opportunities, past as well as present. The opportunity to hear these physicians and to ask questions during these seminars was an important experience for all participants. The rest of this chapter will report in greater detail what we learned from our work with the ten Hampton premedical students.

Some amount of uneasiness developed concerning the success of the summer program during the planning stages in the spring, because of serious student activist unrest and disruption on Cornell's Ithaca campus. These disturbances did not involve Cornell's medical college which is in New York City, except subjectively. Likewise, Hampton Institute was also hit by student activists taking over a building several weeks after the Cornell incident. Plans for the summer program continued despite this turbulence, and the program was assured a favorable start because both at Cornell and at Hampton the collaboration had the support of administration, faculty, and students. Furthermore, while it was known ahead of time that the students would come out of the summer research fellowship experience much more knowledgeable about medicine as a field, and about medical schools, they were given no definite commitment that any certain number of them would be admitted to the medical school. They would of course be urged to apply, not only to Cornell but also to at least five or more other schools, with our advice as to the schools which might be best suited to them. We would also help them to resolve the matter of whether or not medicine was their best career choice. A committee of the Cornell faculty visited the Hampton Institute campus several months ahead of time to meet prospective student applicants and members of the Hampton faculty and administration, and to complete our plans.

Members of the Cornell Medical College faculty had volunteered a number of fellowship projects which they felt would be interesting and challenging, and which the students could handle profitably within the short period of ten weeks. The various departmental offerings were as follows: anatomy had three faculty members whose laboratories had opportunities for one student each; biochemistry had projects for two students; medicine, four students; pathology, two students; pediatrics, three to four students; physiology, one student; pharmacology, two to three students; psychiatry, two students; public health, three to four students. The students were asked to make three choices from these twenty-five offerings, although we realized that they were not able to make very meaningful judgments from their own experience or from the brief paragraphs describing the various projects. Dr. Walter Riker, chairman of the Cornell faculty committee concerned with this program and also head of Cornell's Department of Pharmacology and a long-time faculty member, was largely responsible for deciding on the ten faculty-sponsored projects to be selected. In consultation with me and with Dr. Robert Bonner, the chairman of Hampton's Department of Biology, the students were matched.

We had asked Hampton to send their ten best premedical students. Their faculty were able to locate only twelve students there who were premedical students, and actually only eight seemed certain that they wanted to apply to medical school. As a compromise, we decided to take ten Hampton students. It had seemed that more would be gained by limiting the students to Hampton at least for the first summer, and that the program would include candidates from other colleges in subsequent summers. Moreover, both Cornell and Hampton were strongly motivated to make the program a success. Cornell University Medical College had only two black students in the 1968–1969 year, both African, both planning to return to Africa on completing their medical study. Cornell, like most medical schools, had had only token numbers of Negro students since their first black student graduated in 1915, primarily because strongly qualified applicants had not come forward on their own. Hampton Institute, while ranking fifth among Negro colleges sending students on to medical school, ranked only twelfth among Negro colleges sending students to predominantly white' medical schools. There was no recent memory of a Hampton student submitting application to Cornell's Medical College. We were making a genuine attempt to find and to qualify a group of students who ordinarily would not apply to Cornell, and thus we were increasing our pool of minority group applicants in an immediate sense.

It was our hope that among their best prepared premedical students, at least several might be appropriately admitted. As the students told me later, they knew that efforts were being made to make them feel welcome and comfortable, but they were very much aware that people did not think highly of their ability, because they were black and because they came from a southern black college. Before the summer was over, there had been a great deal of growth in mutual respect as well as friendship. The Hampton students were not only able, but it was clear to all that five of the ten were acceptable candidates for admission to Cornell, and that another two of them were possibly adequate. But the biggest surprise had come to us at the start, from the fact that of Hampton's ten strongest premedical students, six students were blacks from foreign countries and only four were American blacks. Furthermore, the apparent superiority of the foreign black students over the American blacks was the first major finding to understand.

In discussion with Hampton faculty members, it was their impression that although American blacks outnumber foreign blacks by more than a four-to-one ratio at Hampton, the majority of the better premedical students in recent years have been foreigners, although the occasional exceptional student tends to be American. It was also the observation of the Hampton faculty that they had their greatest number of premedical students in the years after World War II. Then as many as forty-five students in one year were premedical, whereas there are currently only about one-third as many. The ten Hampton students divided into three subgroups: (1) the African students, of whom there were three, two from a West African and one from an East African country; (2) the British West Indies students, all three from the same country; and (3) the four Americans, one from the North and three from the South. In fact, the six foreign blacks were sufficiently alike that we can satisfactorily discuss only two groups —the six foreign black students and the four American blacks.

The Six Foreign Students

Similarities in the background of all the foreign students allow us to discuss them as a single group. The two African countries from which the African students came were both former British colonies which gained their independence in 1961, while the British West Indies country had achieved independence from Great Britain in 1967. In all three countries there were many blacks as employees in the civil service, as small businessmen or traders, as well as in the professions. All the foreign students had come from families which had already achieved middle-class status within the civil service or professional job structure of their countries. Usually their parents had been clerks, but two had been teachers. Here was an immediate source of pride. The special boost of having recently achieved national independence made them eager to explain their nation's history, customs, current events, and problems. There was also the pride attached to their family status which set them above the great majority of families in their small countries of origin.

Their early schooling had also been better, and had been attended by feelings of special status. Not everyone went to school in their countries, and most of these students had been able to go only with scholarship support in addition to their parents' earnings. Even their coming to Hampton Institute had been possible for the African students because they were scholarship winners, while the West Indies students had had to spend one or several years earning a sufficient amount to finance their further schooling.

On completing the equivalent of high school, the foreign students spent at least one additional year in each instance in additional study. In the British system, if one completes two additional years of study after the equivalent of our twelfth grade and passes a special examination, he can be admitted to a British university with the equivalent of having completed one and a half years of college credit. If the student completes one or even two such additional years of study and comes to the United States for college, he does not usually receive advanced placement in most American colleges. This was the situation with the foreign Hampton students. They had all begun college study at Hampton as freshmen, although they had at least a year of college-level study in mathematics and in one or another of the sciences such as biology, chemistry, or physics. They therefore had the edge on American freshmen in several ways: they were at least a year older and more mature; they had gained from having had to make the shift to a new country; they had had additional study of science which put them at a competitive advantage. All of them had grade-point averages between "B" and "A" during their Hampton years.

In one interview I asked one of the foreign students to tell me why it was, in his opinion, that there were relatively few American black premedical students. He hesitated at first, and then said, "My views aren't too popular, so I don't have much to say. I don't think Negroes can get what they want just by angry demands, riots, and guns. I think education is the only way."

I agreed essentially, but added that in this country blacks had not had equal educational opportunity.

He smiled and added, "Yes, but on black college campuses the overwhelming majority of students are less than bold in making use of available opportunities to learn. They don't want to work hard, and they avoid the difficult courses. When we [referring to the other foreign students] came to Hampton we found out after a few days that we were the only ones in our class who knew we wanted to be premed students. We talked with the premed advisor [who happens to be the Head of the Chemistry Department], and he advised us all to become chemistry majors because it would give us the strongest premed preparation."[35]

Asked why he thought so few American students choose the more difficult science and math courses, he said, "Well, I think it's because they place emphasis on the wrong things. Many of them come from relatively well-to-do families. They put a lot of emphasis on clothes, external appearances, and on a lot of material things—like how much money you've got. You go to their rooms and you see television, fancy radios, and record players. They go to a lot of parties and are always having a good time, living the life. When you say you're a premed student, they look at you like it's impossible, like you're trying to do the impossible, like trying to shoot for the moon."

"Where," I asked, "do you think some of these differences in attitude come from?"

"I think it's because those of us who come from black countries have an entirely different psychology. When I came here I did not have any feeling of being inferior or unwanted or anything like that, and I didn't know what it meant. It was new to me. I was accustomed to the idea that a black man could be a physician, because all the physicians I had ever seen were black."

He went on to mention that the thirty or so physicians in the town where he lived had gone to school in England, Canada, a few in the United States, and just recently some were coming from the University of the West Indies.

I asked about the way the physicians practice there, "Do they work for the government only, or do they also have private practice, and how much do they earn?"

He answered that they work both in government hospitals and clinics, make visits to outlying rural communities, and also are allowed some private practice. The average physician might earn $12,000 a year, with equal amounts from governmental and from private practice. Although he might be able to buy twice as much for his dollars as an American physician, the American physician earns more. There is also a difference in social status. The few whites who remain in the West Indies are primarily in business or government, while all the professionals—the physicians, lawyers, and teachers, who run all the agencies—are black.

"The life of a physician is very different there from the life of a doctor in America. There a physician is very much admired and respected by everyone wherever he goes. Everyone knows him and looks up to him. He and his family are well cared for."

Another foreign student thought that there were few American premedical students for the following reasons: (1) "They are not told enough about the increased opportunities for admission; many think they could never get in. (2) They don't think they can afford it; they don't know that financial aid is available to them. (3) There are not enough doctors to talk to them, especially black physicians like you, who could come to speak to all the students about medical careers. If there is a speaker, he only speaks to the premed students, or to those who think they may be interested. (4) Few students think of themselves as premeds because in their mind they associate it with being very, very bright, with taking a lot of chem and biology and physics, and with being in school for many years. (5) A lot of students start as biology majors, about eighty in our class as freshmen, but each year a lot of them drop out because they don't like all the hard work. Now there aren't thirty biology majors left in my class, and fewer still will graduate as biology majors. (6) Biology majors are asked to decide during their first year whether they want to go into research, teaching, or medicine. Most of them with the highest grades choose research, but when they get low grades from very hard teachers, they do not change to premed; they drop the biology major completely. They get an inferiority complex about how bright they are."

In fact, at Hampton because the feeling developed that for the prospective premedical student a chemistry major was probably better preparation than a biology major, the Department of Biology began to offer a much more demanding set of courses and teachers, with the result that biology has been losing popularity. It is perhaps true that there is too much specialization in both chemistry and biology majors, and that students are probably groomed for graduate study in one of these fields, rather than for medical school work which would ideally require a broader preparation in science and in non-science areas.

The Four American Students

The American blacks consisted of two who had spent all their lives in small southern urban communities, one who had lived in several different communities in the North and South, and another whose earliest years were spent in the North but who mostly had lived in a southern town. Without exception they had come from families with serious problems of physical or emotional handicap, of struggle for financial security with only marginal job success, except in one instance where a parent was regularly and steadily employed.

Most of them had had all their schooling in segregated school systems, and while they were always among the brightest students in their class, they were not outstanding. At Hampton, which they were not attending as scholarship winners, they were all majoring in biology. It would be erroneous to assume, however, that these students were basically less able than the foreign students. Of the four Hampton students (two African and two American) who had taken the Medical College Admissions Test in May 1969, early enough for us to know their scores during the summer, it was one of the American students whose scores were consistently in the 550 range. His scores were higher than those of any of the other students, although the African student had performed consistently better in the more demanding chemistry major, for reasons which have already been suggested. Generally the American students had between "B" and "C" averages, and had not taken the more rigorous courses in mathematics and chemistry.

The instability in the family structure of American blacks was graphically shown even in so small a number of students, with the weaknesses of fathers being more immediately obvious. This contrasted markedly with the intact, functioning, achievement-oriented and ambitious families of the foreign blacks. The Negro sociologist E. Franklin Frazier,[4] as well as the controversial government official, Daniel Moynihan,[5] have attempted to analyze the causes for this American problem. Ultimately it is tied to the institutionalized role of inferiority for blacks, especially males, which has become a part of the American way of life. Frazier[6] also wrote on the compulsive, frivolous, make-believe fraternity and sorority activities of the American black middle class, which he traced to the lack of real opportunity to play active roles in the mainstream of American society. It should also be remembered that life in the American urbanized and technological culture sets a higher standard for physical, psychiatric, and social competence than is required in less highly developed countries. This may also have made for a poorer showing of the American as compared with the foreign families. The conclusion seemed nonetheless inescapable that the American blacks, while younger and less mature, carried a greater burden of personal and family distress, anxieties about the draft, and uncertainty about the value of a medical career, as well as the grave current climate of alienation which may have been more characteristic of the American youth.

One of the American blacks explained in the following way why there are fewer American than foreign premedical students at Hampton: "I'll tell you why. The American black is an American, and he believes a lot in material things, just like other Americans. He wants everything Whitey has, and he sees himself competing with Whitey to get the same things that Whitey has.

"You take the African black or the West Indies black; he doesn't compare himself with the white man from his country. The few white men there were in a class so far above him that he didn't want to try to get what they had, because it never entered his mind. So the African or West Indies black man is more easily contented and satisfied. He doesn't want as much and he isn't as competitive with Whitey.

"The American black student wants material things, and he wants time to jive around, and he wants time to be with girls and like that. We hang out together because we like the same things: parties, a good time, the same music and dances and that. They, the African and West Indies students, don't like the same kind of music we do, can't do the dances, and don't like to dance with girls that much. So naturally they spend more time with books on weekends. They hang around with each other. Everybody has his own clique at a place like Hampton."

I wondered what, if anything, could be done to make premed more attractive to greater numbers of American blacks.

He admitted, "It won't be easy because of that materialism I was telling you about. The first year after a man graduates from Hampton, he comes back to visit the campus so everybody can see him in his new car, fine clothes, pretty girl if he isn't married, talking about his fine pad and expensive furniture. These are the things he wants and he wants them right away. He doesn't want to wait a whole lot of years while he's going through medical school and internship and all that before he can start making money.

"As soon as he graduates from Hampton he can get a job in industry, if he's a chemistry major, and right away he's making $9,000 or $10,000 a year. Or he goes into a business firm, if he's a business major, making almost the same amount. Within five years they're making a whole lot of money, so they don't see that long medical school. They appreciate they can make a lot if they stick it out, but it seems so long.

"That's why I know I really want it, when I say I want to go to medical school and to be a doctor. I want a car and an apartment right now, real bad, and I still got another year in college. I want it so bad I would be willing to take a job and work, while I'm still trying to graduate from college, but I know I can't do it without lowering my grades and maybe not getting into medical school. I know I can't do it, but I'm tempted.

"A whole lot of white students can have all these things and still go to college and to med school because their folks have a lot of money and can just give it to them. They don't need to worry about things like that."

Another American student had this to add: "There are fewer doctors in those other countries. In this country there are more, so that you might not know there's a shortage of black physicians, especially if you see a lot of them in your city."

She said that she knew perhaps twenty or thirty in the city where she lived. However, she went on to say, "Sometimes knowing black physicians is not a positive experience." When she was small, a private black practitioner who had a reputation of performing tonsillectomies on almost all children he treated, had recommended the operation for her. Her mother checked the recommendation by having her child seen by a white specialist in otolaryngology, who said that there was no need for an operation. He had not known of the other physician's recommendation.

There were more specific complaints from several Hampton students about the inadequacy of the student health service at Hampton, and a realization of the fact that this also had a negative impact on students who might want to be physicians. Hampton is planning to build a hospital and an outpatient clinic, and to provide a much improved health service for students. They already have the money for this new facility, but have not yet begun construction. In the meantime, the infirmary is inadequately staffed by nurses, and by physicians who spend a few hours each day taking care of students' health problems. Students are reluctant to use their services, feeling, as one of them put it, "These physicians were poorly trained and are not the best. Some of them don't know much. We know the reasons. Black physicians didn't have the opportunities when they were coming along that are available now."

Because it is simply a painful and difficult business, the American black students were almost never able to locate very many of their problems within themselves. This was an understandable defensive desire to protect their egos, but it probably served to diminish the demands they might have been able to make on themselves. On the contrary, the foreign students probably had a somewhat too-good picture of themselves. It was clear, however, that this did not at all lower the demands they made on themselves, but rather increased their work output and load.

Evaluating Their Suitability for Medicine

On reviewing the impressions of faculty sponsors, medical and graduate students, and my own impressions gained of the Hampton students in their Seminar course with me, there was a general unanimity of opinion. For two students our impressions at Cornell differed from the impression the Hampton faculty members had forwarded to us. Essentially, we thought one student was less able than they did, and another less interested in medicine, but in all other instances our opinions coincided. The Hampton students were enabled by the summer experience to learn more of medicine, and to judge their suitability and interest in it. As a result, two students decided to enter fields allied to medicine rather than medicine itself (one decided to go into physiotherapy, another into graduate study as a biologist). Of the ten Hampton students, nine applied to Cornell, but one later withdrew his application.

In preparing my report for presentation to the Admissions Committee, I had ranked the Hampton students from first through tenth in terms of my own evaluation of their strength as candidates for admission to Cornell Medical College or a similarly demanding medical school.

The first five, the strongest candidates for admission, were all foreign blacks; all were male; all were chemistry majors; all had had one or more years of scientific study between secondary schooling and their entry at Hampton; all had gradepoint averages of "B" or above. The Admissions Committee members agreed to accept all five of these students, for they had favorably impressed all the Cornell faculty and students who had worked intimately with them during the summer.

The last five, the weaker candidates, contained all four of the American blacks and one foreign student who preferred a field allied to medicine rather than medicine. Both of the girls were in this group. All five of these students were biology majors, and with one exception their grade-point averages were less than "B." My recommendation to the Admissions Committee was that two of these students, both American, were able in my opinion to compete successfully and to complete their studies here at the Cornell Medical School. This opinion was supported for one of the students but there was uncertainty of opinion concerning the other. All were agreed that the three weakest candidates would not, had they wished, have a successful experience as Cornell medical students.

The Admissions Committee, after much deliberation, decided at first to give provisional acceptances to two of the American blacks, with the assurance that if their first semester of senior year work at Hampton raised their average to the level of "B," they would be accepted. One of these students was subsequently accepted, having performed at an exceptionally improved level; the other also improved greatly but elected not to go into medicine.

There was considerable debate and difference of opinion concerning the lack of success of the American blacks in being admitted to the medical school, but the view prevailed that an unfortunate trail of hardship and turmoil would have accompanied their admission into a situation of almost certain failure. Even so, some of us were made more acutely aware than ever that the entire lifetime of environmental deprivation in America was not the personal responsibility of these individual American blacks or their families, but rather more accurately represented a failure of the whole American community. The superior performance profiles of the foreign blacks, despite the fact of their origin in underdeveloped countries weak in total resources, pointed to the obvious connections between educational and emotional and community input, and subsequent academic achievement. Both success and failure tend to become self-perpetuating, as we had observed, but we could also notice that the special summer program did bring about important attitude change in several Hampton students.

Quotas and Standards

The medical manpower recruitment process in this country has had the unfortunate result of selecting too many whites from high-income families, a process which can be expected to accelerate with the rapidly rising costs of medical and other higher education. This is the most obvious reason that simply doubling the number of medical students in schools might make no dent at all in the shortage of physicians taking care of a cross-section of the American public. Unless special programs are started, only the wealthy family will be able to send a child to medical school. Simultaneously, we are as a nation for the first time attempting, and promising, to deliver high-quality health care to the whole American community, to people of all social and income levels. This will never happen unless all social groups are trained at all levels of the health system, for all groups must take part in planning, exploring, and implementing this new system of health delivery. Since the medical schools can educate only limited numbers of physicians, it would follow that medical schools will be required to use quota systems of some kind to allow greater representation of previously underrepresented minority groups in our medical schools. These previously excluded groups are blacks, Spanish-surnamed Americans, American Indians, women, and all white Americans who are among the thirty million citizens who live in poverty.

The process of their entry into medical schools will be smoother if prospective medical school candidates from those groups are identified at high school or college levels, and brought up to competitive parity with students who appear more able because of more privileged educational backgrounds.

Many will be concerned that standards may be lowered or sacrificed, but such anxieties cannot obscure the obvious fact that large numbers of highly intelligent American youth have simply been excluded from first-class educational opportunities. This can be remedied with relative ease, if conscious efforts are directed toward that end. The privileged groups, on the other hand, have enjoyed not only increasing material resources but increasing educational resources as well, as is reflected in the gradual increase in MCAT scores, between 50 and 75 points in the four categories, with the average scores beginning to more into the 600 range. The educational opportunity gulf is widening, and such disparities are always more evident at graduate and professional school educational levels. Since our technological scientific world has opened up jobs for more highly educated and highly intelligent people than ever before, we must reshape educational policies concerning admissions, as well as in other ways, in order to produce these new professionals and scientists.

Grade-point averages for students accepted by medical schools have generally shown in the past decade or so that about fifteen percent have an "A" average, ten percent have a "C" average, and the overwhelming majority, or around seventy-five percent, are "B" students. Since grades from different colleges are not easily translated into equivalents of actual preparation, the MCAT test was an attempt to judge the amount of achieved quality learning in verbal, quantitative thinking, general information, and science areas. Few would doubt that the MCAT favors students who have been well taught in the best schools. Statistically this means it has favored well educated, high-income, white families. Grade-point averages are often considered a more stable index of a student's overall abilities to organize his time, to study and learn; and the subjects in which he does the best work are generally thought to show his genuine interests as well as his ability. It is also generally conceded that MCAT scores and gpa's are more predictive of success in the first two years of medical school, the basic science years; and are less predictive of the last two clinical years of medical school, still less predictive of the physician's effectiveness as an intern or resident, and still less predictive of his success or competence or contribution as a career physician. This being so, there is little convincing basis for rigid insistence on absolute cut-off points on the MCAT or grade-point average.[7]

Common sense as well as flexibility would argue strongly, however, in favor of accepting minority group students whose average MCAT scores are as close to the 500 to 600 level as possible, and that their grade-point averages should remain as close to the general distribution of "A," "B," and "C" averages as possible. The students must remain within the same academic program as other students, graded and evaluated in the same format, if any genuine classroom integration is to occur. On the same reasoning, if the medical schools genuinely believe in the meaning of such performance measure as MCAT's and gpa's, they can, at a reasonable expenditure of their resources, identify minority youngsters at college and high school levels and influence their educational opportunity sufficiently to bring them to levels of competitive parity. This would set a new standard of socially responsive behavior on the part of the medical profession, and the medical educational system, which would provide leadership for the more sluggish and unresponsive bureaucracies.

Summary

In the summer of 1969 Cornell University Medical College, in response to growing conviction of the important need for active recruitment of able black premedical students, provided its first ten-week summer research fellowship for minority group students. The program was conducted collaboratively with one predominantly black college, Hampton Institute in Virginia. Hampton was asked to send their ten best premedical students who had completed their junior year, and who would ordinarily be at the point of applying to medical schools.

The research fellowship was under the guidance and sponsorship of individual faculty members of the medical school, but the Hampton students worked closely with medical students and predoctoral students in the Graduate School of Medical Science who held similar summer fellowships.

Seminars, twice weekly, were designed to help the student become aware of the varieties of medical careers, of the particular expansion in opportunity for the prospective black physician, and the students were given specific introduction to the nature of medical school studies, the process of applying to medical school and obtaining financial aid.

The ten Hampton students presented several interesting features; for one, the five chemistry majors seemed to have a more complete and rigorous scientific preparation for medical study than the five biology majors.

The ten Hampton students came from different parts of the world: three were from Africa; three were from the British West Indies, and only four were from the United States. The foreign students were different in other ways: They were slightly older, had had at least an additional year of science studies, were usually chemistry majors, had earlier and firmer decisions to be premedical students. They also had stronger and more supportive family backgrounds, as well as a more positive image of the physician and of a medical career.

Some of the attitudes of foreign and American black premedical students are presented and their meanings explored.

Programs to recruit American blacks into the field of medicine will require much more careful and special support, starting in earlier years, because of special disabilities and deprivations which have been inherent in the cultural situation of American blacks.

The potential contribution to American medical manpower of potentially able American black youth warrants these special efforts.

Special collaborative programs of medical schools working with black premedical students can be rewarding mutual learning experiences, and are run with relative ease, provided they have the support of administration, faculty and students as was true in this instance.

V

Impact on the
Medical Schools (1969)

The New York Metropolitan
Area Medical Schools

The Report of New York State to the U.S. Civil Rights Commission revealed that in the year 1963–1964 there were only seventeen Negro students in the first-year classes of the six local medical colleges.[1] Even this figure of seventeen may be an overestimation, as it was at times a guess based on looking at a photograph, not to mention the fact that a very large proportion of these Negro students must have been from foreign countries. Cornell itself, for example, graduated only two American blacks from 1960 through 1969, and they graduated two blacks from other countries during that same decade.

This pattern of slowness of change was transformed into noticeable movement within two years. In 1968 each of the seven medical schools in the New York City area designated one of their deans or a member of their Admissions Committee to meet regularly, at least once monthly, to share common concerns, resources, and procedures, and to avoid wasteful duplication of effort in their programs to attract promising black applicants to their schools. Thus the Metropolitan Committee for

Minority Groups in Medicine was formed. The schools observed repeatedly that several of them would send out acceptances to the same small number of qualified black students, who might not end up attending any one of the metropolitan schools. It graphically pointed to the need of plans to enlarge the pool of "qualified applicants," a term which rankles the feelings of many. In fact, and I believe with good reason, the schools are seeking the most highly qualified black applicants they can find. Beyond that, each school was also actually operating or planning a program to enlarge the pool of applicants who would be able to compete successfully with their other students. Briefly these programs, as of the spring of 1969, were as follows:[2]

1. The Cornell University Medical college program which was discussed in the preceding chapter.

2. Mt. Sinai School of Medicine sent staff members on visits to a number of predominantly black colleges to recruit applicants. In addition, because their medical school is a part of the New York City University, they made a special effort to work with the SEEK and College Discovery programs in the undergraduate colleges to find promising students and to arrange work-study programs at the medical school on an individualized basis.

3. The New York Medical College faculty and students established its "Med-Start" program to interest high school students in the medical field, and had begun to explore a possible program with Harlem Prep, the well-known street academy program for high school drop-outs, many of whom go on to college. Students and faculty were also involved in recruitment as well as medical college admissions interviewing of minority group candidates. They were also seeking sources of financial support.

4. Columbia students particularly were pushing for active recruitment, scholarships for those admitted, special educational and tutoring programs, all of which the university generally supported. Efforts were made to locate college premeds and high school students, locally as well as in southern colleges. Liaison was being developed with their parent university's School of General Studies and the newly established Urban Center for the initiation of other programs.

5. Albert Einstein College of Medicine of Yeshiva University instituted a special supplementary premedical year, known as the "Martin Luther King—Robert F. Kennedy Program for Special Studies at the Albert Einstein College of Medicine." Applicants were chosen with the cooperation and suggestion of premedical advisors in the colleges, as well as of their own faculty members and staff. The seven scholarship winners selected spent their year pursuing a special curriculum of study (organic chemistry, cell biology, mathematics, etc.) designed to strengthen their premedical preparation, and they were allowed to audit selected first-year courses at the medical school. They were also paid a stipend to cover living expenses.

6. New York University established a special faculty-student subcommittee of the Admissions Committee to develop a program of active recruitment, to establish contact with black and other minority group premedical students and their advisors, and to interview minority group applicants who were to be given financial aid as required.

7. State University of New York at Downstate Medical Center, in collaboration with Brooklyn College, initiated a program for the early identification of minority group students who showed promise for medical careers despite some academic difficulty resulting from poor earlier schooling. These students were given special guidance, counseling, tutoring, financial aid, and the chance of being accepted into the medical school on completion of the premedical studies at Brooklyn College. Faculty and student committees also are involved in contacting potential premedical students at college and at high school levels to foster and strengthen medical career interest, provide opportunities for summer research study and work.

Moreover, all of this activity was producing results, as is shown from the numbers of black students entering the first-year classes of these schools in the 1969–1970 year: Cornell (2), Mt. Sinai (4), New York Medical College (8), Columbia (7), Albert Einstein (14), New York University (6), State University of New York at Downstate Medical Center (4). Thus in one year a total of 45 black students were actually enrolled, representing 5.3% of all the 846 first-year students enrolled in these medical schools. This was a severalfold increase over 1963–1964, and represented the first significant increase in black student enrollment in New York metropolitan area medical schools.

But this still is not an adequate response to the medical manpower needs of the New York City area where fourteen percent of the population is black and approximately eight percent is Puerto Rican. The one quarter of the city's minority population is still grossly under-represented in the local area medical student population, local schools having been slightly at or below the national two percent average for many years. Nor did it seem that the problem was to be solved by any immediate program. In the fall of 1969–1970 a subcommittee of the Metropolitan Committee for Minority Groups in Medicine established, after polling the premedical advisors in local undergraduate colleges, that only fifty to one hundred black or Puerto Rican students attending these colleges were known to be premedical students, counting all freshmen, sophomores, juniors and seniors combined. This alarming scarcity exists despite the fact that over half of all children attending New York City public schools are black or Puerto Rican. Only a few years ago less than ten percent of the students enrolled in regular four-year colleges of the City University of New York were black or Puerto Rican. It was another gross indication that a separate system of special, parochial, private, and suburban secondary schools are the chief suppliers of premedical students to our metropolitan area and other colleges. It is a show of pathetic failure of our public school system for minority group children.

Accordingly the Metropolitan Committee began to work directly with high school guidance counselors at the senior academic high school level, particularly with youngsters who show potential for college-level and professional school work. The premedical advisors from local colleges are working together with some of us from the medical schools, since we are well aware that any effective program must bridge the high school, college, and medical school years. We confidently expect that within a few years large numbers of able and well-qualified black and Puerto Rican premedical students will be applying for admission to the medical schools, not only here in the New York metropolitan area, but in all parts of the country.

Impact on Cornell's Admission Policy

It will be recalled that for the class which entered in the fall of 1969, Cornell Medical School had two black freshmen, which represented a small fraction of their total class of eighty-nine students. The increase was a distinct and definite one, and since both of these stu-

dents were American blacks, it represented more than
had been present in any class during at least the preceding decade. However, it raised the question as to
whether Cornell's admissions policy was still too restric-
tive, compared with other schools. For that year, the
students and faculty had increased significantly the
number of blacks who applied to Cornell; there were
twenty-five applicants in all, several times the usual
number. Moreover, places had been offered to six, but
four elected not to come.

The author made a follow-up study of all twenty-
five applicants, in the late fall and early winter of 1969.
Of the four accepted applicants who did not choose to
come to Cornell, one decided to spend a year in travel
and study, but the three others elected other medical
schools (Yale, N.Y.U., Tufts). One of the other nineteen
students had been put on the waiting list, or in other
words had been given a provisional acceptance depend-
ing on whether or not a place became available. That
student had been accepted by Harvard and was enrolled there.

Another three withdrew their applications before
Cornell had taken final action. Two of these had gone
to Harvard, the other had gone to Stanford.

The remaining fifteen had been rejected by Cornell. Only one of these failed to get into any medical
school. One is attending the graduate school of medical
science at a medical school, working on a Ph.D. in biochemistry. All the other thirteen are attending predominantly white medical schools (specifically these schools
are: Columbia, Einstein, University of Chicago, Wayne
State, University of Pittsburgh, State University of New
York Upstate and Downstate, University of California).
This follow-up study did indeed suggest that Cornell's
admission procedures were not as receptive to black
applicants as some of the other leading schools.

Other Aspects of the Impact of Black Enrollment On New York City Area Medical Schools

Concerning other aspects of the impact on the medical schools in the New York City area we can make the following observations. Uniformly all the schools took part in the process of desegregating their schools as a response to widespread student and faculty sentiment that such a change should be made. This was almost certainly a response to the fact that all the nation's leading schools had made similar policy changes. Schools in the New York City area furthermore found uniformly that as they increased their underrepresented minority enrollment, it made increased demands on their funds for student financial aid, since most of these students required more than previously registered levels of financial need. The schools in the New York City area also seemed generally persuaded of the wisdom of admitting to medical school only those students who would be able to pursue their standard medical school curriculum and their standard system of grading and evaluation. All the schools were moving toward increasing the amount of free or elective time beginning in the first year of medical school, and toward a system of earlier introduction of clinically relevant medical knowledge and study of health care delivery systems, as well as plans to adopt a pass, pass-with-honors, and fail system of grading. All of these changes were being made out of a response to pressure from students and faculty to upgrade the general quality of medical education for all students, rather than a specific accommodation to the needs of black students. In other words, it was our thinking generally, and certainly at Cornell, that a sound educational policy and program would be suitable for all students, whose individual needs for guidance and advice would not be accurately gauged by skin color.

Impact on Black Medical Schools

The nationwide search for the best qualified black applicants to medical schools was not without significant impact on Howard and Meharry, the two predominantly black medical schools. It will be recalled that since the late 1940's proponents of civil rights for Negroes had concluded that it would be in the best interests of Negroes generally, of Howard and Meharry, and of the public health of the nation at large, if segregated education were abolished. This would not at all necessarily mean abolishing Howard and Meharry, but rather that all the nation's medical schools would admit black and white applicants, and adopt a uniform admissions policy which would not be racially exclusive. The fundamental logic of this point of view, that as a nation we should have a single and uniform, racially inclusive rather than racially exclusive admissions policy, is in my opinion unassailable. In short, we should complete the process of doing away with racially segregated schools. For many years Howard University, which was financed by the federal government, admitted only token numbers of whites, only a few per class, although in recent years they reached a white enrollment of approximately twenty-five percent. The Howard University School of Dentistry has gone much further along the lines of racial integration and in recent years over sixty percent of their student body has been white. The results for the Howard School of Dentistry were in the direction predicted by long-time civil rights proponents: the Howard School of Dentistry has become a stronger school, with a more qualified and able student body and with a strengthened faculty and program.

These changes in the School of Dentistry were forced as a result of reduced black applications when admissions opportunities increased for blacks at the predominantly white dental schools. Also, having achieved much of this change a few years earlier, the School of Dentistry at Howard was able to escape the militant racial polarization which had become more intense within the past two years.

We can follow the events at Howard in greater detail because of the associated turbulence, which was reported in the Negro press, and which has been discussed by the author with several members of the Howard alumni, faculty, students, and some of the newspapermen who covered these developments.

Of the class of one hundred entering Howard in the fall of 1968, thirteen students were white. Several classes had had even greater numbers of white students, but perhaps already in that year there was a beginning of increased feelings of racial animosity. The anti-white revolutionary rhetoric of the black student activists, so much a feature at Howard, the leading Negro university in this country, was bound to have an effect on their medical school student body. The white students in that class found that several Negro students were friendly and helpful in giving them a feeling of welcome and security, but another few Negro students were openly hostile, while the rest played the role of the usual silent majority. There were many demands for curriculum reform and for generally improved educational policy and practice were similar to those heard at other medical schools. These demands began to take on a different tone.

For the class entering Howard in the fall of 1969, a much more difficult problem arose. With places for approximately one hundred and five in the first-year class, only eighty-three students showed up for registration, leaving the school about twenty-two students short of a complete class. Among the students who appeared on the day of registration were the twenty-three whites who had been accepted, and there were a number of other white applicants on the waiting list who would have enrolled if given the chance. A number of black students, in other words, had been accepted by Howard and by one or several predominantly white schools as well, and had inexcusably not notified Howard that they would not be coming there.

It was not only that Howard does not have the prestige, faculty, program or other facilities that the other schools have to offer; it was also a fact that over the years Howard's school costs were lower than those at the predominantly white schools, and for this reason they had attracted a number of able black students who might have elected to go elsewhere. With the white schools admitting Negroes and taking care of their financial needs as well, Howard and Meharry lost the competitive advantage of their lower costs. They did not have scholarships which were competitive. In my opinion, the clear gain was to the students who went to stronger schools. They will profit by a fuller development of their potential as physicians, as will all the institutions and persons who will use their future services.

At that point the black student activists at Howard threatened to close the medical school if more than twenty-three whites were admitted to the class entering in 1969, insisting that only black students be admitted from the waiting list. They also began to make overt claims that Howard was, and should become even more completely, a black medical school, that there should be practically an open admissions policy for any black student applying to Howard; that practically any black student admitted should also be graduated. There was the definite statement that the white student quota should be reduced to a very small number indeed, and there should be a considerable expansion in black enrollment. Ultimately Howard was able to enroll only ninety-eight students for a class which should have contained one hundred and five.

This militant ideology also maintained not only that white students at Howard were taking places away from blacks, but that white graduates of Howard would have no further interest either in the school or in black patients after graduation, that whites and blacks have no common basis for working with or understanding each other. More and more the white students found themselves emotionally cut off from ordinary friendly conversations or collaboration, and the atmosphere became racially oppressive. Many white students made unsuccessful efforts to transfer to other schools, the atmosphere had become so unconducive to medical study and learning.

We were observing more than a black militant demand for a separate black institution; we were also hearing an insistence on dual and separate standards or measures of competence. If any black who applies to medical school must be accepted on a first-come, first-served basis, with his blackness and his desire to study medicine his only admission requirement, assuming legal requirements are met, we should in no time at all produce another category of third-rate physicians. If in addition to totally open admissions we have also a grading system for such students consisting of an automatic "pass," with no grade of "honors" or "fail," almost all institutionalized support or incentive for effective teaching or learning would be removed. The graduate of such a medical school would not possibly be considered a colleague by graduates of other medical schools. The only conceivable way in which such a total revolution in the admissions, grading, and graduation of students could begin, granting it might be considered socially responsible enough to be considered an experimental educational scheme, would be for it to be tried by one or two of those medical schools with long established positions and traditions of standard academic excellence. In any event it seems clear that if the proposed double standard put forward by these few black student militants were to be adopted at Howard, admission to and graduation from the medical school would become entirely a matter of what family had the greatest amount of political muscle to force entry of his child into the medical profession. We have already had enough of the appearance, if not the actuality, of that kind of unhealthy and unfair control of the medical educational apparatus in this country. Moreover, it is an abject surrender to racial segregation and second-class citizenship of a reactionary rather than revolutionary thrust.

Going beyond the matter of separate black schools, with separate standards of admissions and graduation, is the assumption that black physicians will only work with black patients, for it follows that if whites cannot work with or understand blacks the converse must also be true. The matter escalated higher still, until there were assertions that a white psychiatrist on the faculty could not teach black students anything about a psychiatric disorder such as schizophrenia. The basic metabolic disturbances which apparently underlie the schizophrenic disease process, and the psychopathologic disturbances which are known to occur in schizophrenics of all ethnic and social class groups, are given modified expressions in various cultural or subcultural settings, but there is not the slimmest evidence that diagnosis or treatment or rehabilitation can be based on a patient's skin color or racial identity. The black student minority claimed that because blacks have suffered through four hundred years of slavery, this has made their minds, mentalities, and personalities inscrutable and impenetrable to all whites. As a psychiatrist, I should like to point out in passing that schizophrenic patients in particular, but by no means exclusively, commonly feel that they are worthless, inferior, different, damaged, downtrodden, misunderstood, and past all hope of meaningful human contact and interchange. I have seen patients with these feelings, I should add, from the most highly privileged social and ethnic groups, some of whom as individuals were even of outstanding potential and attainment. So vehement was the shrill insistence that a white cannot teach psychiatry to blacks, that one white faculty member at Howard resigned, after noting that the attitude did not moderate.

It should be borne in mind that even in those medical diseases, such as sickle cell anemia, known to occur almost exclusively in blacks and only rarely in whites, the challenge to understand and gain control over this disorder is not a problem for blacks only to understand and to solve. Within the past two decades considerable progress has been made in understanding and treating sickle cell anemia, but the medical scientists who have been drawn to this field have come from those medical schools and universities with the most powerful resources for research. Howard and Meharry have not been the medical centers which have taken the lead in the study of this disease, nor should they feel compelled to divert their resources disproportionately to the study of only one of the diseases from which their black patients and other patients will suffer. The fundamental fact that the human race consists of only one species is the biological basis for the philosophical doctrine of the brotherhood of man, and is the driving force toward the creation of a unified, worldwide human sense of community. Most observers are convinced that the overwhelming majority point of view among the faculty and student bodies at Howard and Meharry rejects the racial separatist philosophy.

Reitzes pointed out in his survey of fourteen major U.S. communities that the extent to which Negro professionals were integrated into the medical structure and opportunity hierarchy was related to the presence

and importance of Negro hospitals which served to produce self-segregation, isolation, and acceptance of the
status quo.[3] In communities where influential persons
and groups maintained steady and constant pressure for
integration, and where Negro physicians made sacrifices
to upgrade their professional skills, the integration process was furthered—a process which had every likelihood of continuing in view of the shortage of physicians, interns, residents, and salaried hospital staff.
Decades earlier, Negro leaders generally opposed the
building of Negro hospitals in Negro ghettoes of large
northern cities, and had instead pressed for the admission of Negroes to general municipal hospitals serving
everybody in the community. A similar logic had led
Negro leadership to oppose the establishment of large
Veterans Administration hospitals at Howard University and Meharry, because this superstructure would
only have delayed their eventual integration into a single system of medical education and health care in decades to come (Cobb 1947).[4] The decade for integration
to have come, but the process is far from smooth.

Summary

Reviewing the impact of the move to desegregate medical schools in the United States, we first directed attention to the seven schools in the metropolitan New York
City area. For some years less than two percent of the
student bodies of the New York City area schools had
been black, but there was a more than doubling of black
enrollment in the classes which entered in the fall of
1969. The collaborative efforts of the New York City
medical schools, through the Metropolitan Committee
for Minority Groups in Medicine, will be aimed at working with the area high school, premedical college, as
well as medical school level, for only in this way will a
greater supply of qualified black applicants become

available. Cornell's admissions policy showed a change in acceptance of black applicants.

The talent search for qualified black applicants to all the medical schools will predictably produce a painful impact on the predominately black medical schools, which must rapidly undergo favorable or unfavorable change. For many years the civil rights movement for American blacks had maintained that as all the nation's medical schools dropped their color barriers, Howard and Meharry would become stronger schools by simultaneously welcoming white as well as black students on as close to a single standard as possible. Racial inclusiveness rather than racial exclusiveness would have a favorable effect on the medical education of all physicians and on their future careers as deliverers of health services.

There are indications that the black medical schools will have increasing difficulty attracting those black applicants who are best qualified, under current criteria, as future physicians. This is true of black colleges generally as well.

This has given rise to a black militant separatist faction who speak for perpetuation of dual standards for admission and graduation of black students to black schools specifically aimed at producing blacks who will work only with black patients.

A historical heritage of racial segregation and separatism would account for such opinions, along with the fact that segregated institutions, white or black, resist change.

VI

Impact on the
Medical Schools (1970)

Black Enrollment at Cornell in 1970

I was able to report to the Executive Faculty, shortly
after the beginning of the 1970–1971 school year, that
of the ninety-one newly enrolled freshmen at Cornell
ten were black and two Puerto Rican. Since we had one
black student in his fourth year, and another in his second, and no Puerto Ricans, the total minority enrollment at Cornell was still not great when we consider
that there are about three hundred and sixty students
in all. It was with some discomfort that I reported that
of the two black students accepted at Cornell last year,
one fared poorly here, and is repeating the first year at
another medical school. Despite this, I felt certain that
the minority group students we admitted were not only
able, but were capable of becoming outstanding future
physicians.

The newly enrolled minority group students presented a fortunate range of diversity in background:
two were from West Africa, three were from the West
Indies, five were American blacks, and two were American Puerto Ricans. In every way conceivable it was my
aim to see that these students were treated as individuals, as all students should be treated, and that they

were protected against pressures to lump them together into one group.

A total of ninety-five blacks applied to Cornell last year; fifteen were accepted, and ten are currently enrolled. Of the five who went elsewhere, three preferred Harvard and two preferred the University of Pennsylvania. Pennsylvania impressed both these students because a year or so earlier that university had begun to enroll greater numbers of black students, and its medical center was actively involved in experimental health care delivery programs in the ghetto neighborhood. The two students who selected Pennsylvania were also our only black applicants who were from financially independent families, able to pay their own way completely. It should be noted at this point, however, that all the black applicants, regardless of means, were genuinely driven to devote their professional lives to their less fortunate brethren, quite unbelievable as that may sound. I cannot too strongly stress the fact that black and Puerto Rican medical students really believe what they are saying and planning to do with their future lives. This dedication to the welfare of their fellow man is a new phenomenon for those of us who, even though highly altruistic, grew up in earlier decades.

In any event, the minority group students accepted at Cornell were still in 1970 very carefully chosen, as can be seen from the fact that Harvard accepted two students who were not accepted at Cornell. We should also note the extreme scarcity of Puerto Rican applicants. There were only four, of whom we accepted two. They were, nonetheless, in every way well prepared graduates of CCNY and Brooklyn College, respectively. The black students had come from the following schools: six from Hampton and one each from Hobart, American University in Washington, D.C., Brooklyn College, and C. W. Post. Clearly these students were an excellent sample of the minority groups throughout the nation. From one year to the next a major change had taken place in opening up the Cornell Medical College to minority group students.

Black Enrollment at Medical Schools in the New York City Metropolitan Area

It will be recalled that in the New York City area, 1969 was indeed the first year that local area medical schools had admitted more than token numbers of minority group students. In that year, forty-five minority group students had been among the eight hundred and forty-six admitted to first-year classes by the seven New York City metropolitan schools. This represented, nonetheless, 5.3% of all first-year medical students, which put New York City ahead of the 2.75% enrollment of minority group students in the nation as a whole in that year.

Since many of us were uncertain of our progress during the year, it was with some feeling of relief and satisfaction that we found a progressively improving admissions situation in the New York City area schools in the fall of 1970. The combined first-year class enrollments for the seven schools consisted of eight hundred and sixty-seven students, of whom seventy were from minority groups—sixty-two blacks and eight Puerto Ricans. This represented eight percent of first-year enrolled medical students. Considering that New York City is fourteen percent black and eight percent Puerto Rican, we should, of course, aim at higher levels of enrollment than the twelve percent nationwide target set by the AAMC Task Force report previously mentioned. At the annual meeting of the AAMC in the fall of 1970 it was announced that minority-group students, almost all blacks, were 697 of all entering freshmen, which comprised 6.1 percent of the entering class for that year nationwide. It will be seen that the New York City area schools slightly exceeded this nationwide percentage.

Compared to the first-year enrollments of the other New York City area medical schools in 1970, Cornell's 13.1% of black and Puerto Rican students exceeded all the other local medical schools this year. Since Columbia began its recruitment program more vigorously last year, it slightly exceeds Cornell in overall minority group student enrollment.

Specifically the schools made the following achievements: Cornell with an entering class of ninety-one enrolled ten blacks and two Puerto Ricans; Columbia with a class of one hundred and thirty-eight had fifteen black freshmen; Einstein with a class of one hundred and fifteen had seven blacks and three Puerto Ricans; SUNY Downstate with a class of two hundred and five enrolled seventeen blacks and one Puerto Rican; New York University with a freshman class of one hundred and forty enrolled eight blacks; Mt. Sinai with a class of forty enrolled three blacks and one Puerto Rican; and New York Medical College with a class of one hundred and thirty-eight admitted only two blacks and one Puerto Rican.

The New York Medical College situation was certainly a painful one for a number of persons. In 1969, they had admitted seven blacks and one Puerto Rican, most of whom had been out of school and pursuing other professional work, but were highly motivated to enter medical school. Five of those students were being asked to repeat the year because their performance had not been up to usual standards. This performance caused a number of persons to question the validity of admitting greater numbers of minority students to that school unless arrangements for providing extra, and expensive, remedial programs were also made. The reduced number of students accepted in 1970 reflected the small number of minority group students who would not require special or separate programs there.

Considerable difficulty had also been experienced by the fourteen minority group students who had entered Einstein in 1969. Only four of them had turned in really satisfactory performances; while of the remaining ten, three were advanced to the second year with the requirement of passing make-up exams. One is taking the whole year over, and the remaining six performed so poorly that they may require an additional year or more to complete medical school, if they are able to do so at all. Here too there was a realization from the start that students had been admitted who, although they had a great deal of potential and motivation, lacked standard academic achievement profiles. The reduced number of minority admissions to Einstein in 1970 probably was at least partly a response to the extremely uneven level of performance of these minority group students.

Having experienced at first hand the task of advising one of the two black freshmen enrolled at Cornell in 1969 to repeat the year at another school, I know how much trauma and heartbreak are involved for students who are not able to compete successfully with their classmates. Experiences of this kind are extremely valuable for anyone who would take lightly the matter of matching the best medical school with a particular student. While this process, a dynamic and ever-changing one, cannot be captured in an easy formula, it is at the very least a decision requiring great care and thought. Particularly for the black, Puerto Rican, or other minority group student, it is as true as it has always been that it is much sounder to go first to the appropriate medical school than to gamble on being able to transfer later. Transfers from one medical school to another, or a flexible extension of the number of years until graduation, are not a part of standard operating procedure at this time. Too much, however, can be made of a mistaken admission decision. If a school has no students who do poorly, it should suggest that the admissions criteria are too rigid and cautious, and that conservatism or conventionality are perhaps being too much rewarded.

These were some of the preoccupations and concerns at the various medical schools, and those of us who had come to know each other through our regular meetings of the Metropolitan Committee for Minority Groups in Medicine were convinced that our schools could only learn to become more expert in meeting the needs of minority group students by admitting these students. While there is no necessity to give further detail, all the schools found that their minority group students, as a whole, had not done as well scholastically as the rest of their class. We were all continuing our search for those programs which would help us more accurately to accept potentially successful students. At the same time we were committed to the need to identify and select able students at secondary school and college level, and to stregthen their interests in medicine.

Summer Research and Other
Summer Programs at Cornell

A. Summer Jobs at the Medical Center

We realized that some means should be found of bringing to the Cornell Medical Center a number of minority group premedical students, particularly during the crucial first two years when so many of them abandon plans for a medical career. Thus, they would gain employment and clarify their career goals at the same time. Through the kindness of the Departments of Nursing at the New York Hospital, the Payne Whitney Clinic, the Westchester Division of Payne Whitney, and the Burke Rehabilitation Center, we were able to provide summer vacation employment for twenty-eight college students, twenty-four black and four Puerto Rican. These students earned $105 per week, were given training, and worked under supervision as ward clerks or nurses' aides. They functioned extremely well in these roles. All of them attended colleges or universities in the northeastern United States and lived in the New York City area, so that they were able to commute from home to work. I had come to know these students in a variety of ways, but it provided an excellent opportunity always for me to become acquainted with the premedical advisors at their schools, and to hear from them what problems they were discovering. One of these students was just entering college; eighteen had completed the first year; two had completed the second year; five had finished the junior year, and the remaining two had finished college and were to begin medical school here in the fall. From this distribution, there is a strong indication that a great number of students stop thinking of a medical career after the first or second year of extremely difficult work. These students came from the following schools: six from Cornell University, five from Williams College, three from Brooklyn College, two from Queens College, two from State University at Stonybrook, and one each from Columbia, CCNY, Long Island University, Fisk, Vassar, Barnard, C. W. Post, NYU, and Syracuse University.

It was our plan that through the individual and group support, as well as informal friendship and guidance, that these students would receive by coming to know a number of helpful persons here, we would contribute to their preparation as premedical students. For three students, by the end of the summer, it did seem that medicine would not be a good career choice, because they seemed to lack ability, interest, motivation, maturity or the ability to accept reasonable supervision. Here again, these qualities are only gradually learned.

Summer employment is hard to find, especially for minority group students, and many of these people would have been forced to accept employment of an extremely menial nature. Some of them had actually worked as kitchen helpers in a hospital, as stock clerks, had pushed a cart in the garment district, and done factory work—to name actual jobs some of them had held.

B. Summer Research Fellowships Continued

The foregoing program was in addition to the summer research fellowships we had begun in the summer of 1969 with the ten Hampton students. In fact, the six Hampton students who had been accepted to enter Cornell in the fall of 1970 were invited to return in the summer of 1970 for a second summer. They were already accepted into the medical school and knew their way around, and because they did not attend again the seminars on the various medical career fields and specialties, they had more time for individual research work or study. Some of the excitement had worn off, as well as some of the anxiety, and several of the Hampton students felt that they might have enjoyed a job as a laboratory assistant or a nurse's aide or ward clerk, rather than the greater amount of independent effort that was involved in trying to complete even a small research project in a ten-week period. On the other hand, none of them could have known exactly how they would have spent a more profitable summer before entering medical school.

For the summer of 1970 we had a new group of sixteen post-junior-year premedical students from a variety of colleges and universities: four from Queens College, three from Cornell University, two from CCNY, two from Columbia University, two from Hampton Institute, and one each from Brooklyn College, Hofstra University, and York College. Of the sixteen, we had fifteen American blacks and one Puerto Rican; twelve were male and four female; fourteen were single and two were married. All were with us for a ten-week period, receiving $100-a-week stipends to cover expenses, and all single students lived in the medical students' dormitory. Of course, the major difference between this group and that of the preceding summer was the fact that the second group was almost completely made up of American blacks from a number of different schools rather than one. We knew this would make the group experience a different one, but we were really not sure in what way.

Our aims for this group were essentially the same as the previous year, except that we wanted these students to learn more about the medical school curriculum, the faculty-student atmosphere, the medical center's interest in health care delivery, its strengths in the basic sciences, and their relevance to medicine. In the course of the summer, the students would get a clearer picture of whether Cornell was the school for them, and a number of faculty, students, and administration personnel could have a basis for opinions as to their probable strength as students. The format included the twice-weekly seminars in which the sixteen met with me and heard about special career fields in the basic and clinical sciences and of current developments and opportunities in the various fields. As their major activity, of course, they also had the independent research assignment to a faculty member engaged in research activities, with the aim of allowing each student to do as much independent work as feasible.

New features were added in an effort to bring greater pertinence to this exploratory ten-week stay with us. They were potential students who would be with us for several years, not prospective research scientists. For that reason we decided to include a special introductory physiology course, planned by Dr. Walter Riker, Professor of Pharmacology and a close colleague of mine in the entire program. The course was to be held twice weekly with two-hour sessions taught by volunteers among medical students and students of our Graduate School of Medical Sciences. Summer Fellows were to be given a brief course at the level of medical school work, as a preview of what classwork in a basic science is like. Additionally, each Fellow was assigned to a third-year medical student volunteer, who agreed to meet regularly with the students to take them to the wards, and introduce them to clinical work with sick patients, the kind of clinical learning that is the core of the last two years of medical school. We were able to offer this part of the program because third-year medical students are normally present and their class is in session until August. Without exception, the minority group students were enthusiastic about this early introduction to clinical work, and more than anything else it convinced them that they could anticipate becoming a part of the medical team in this institution. Few of them had really believed it at the beginning of the summer. They had to have the actual experience of being well received, of not encountering race prejudice or insult, before they could believe it possible. This had a definite effect on the staff of the hospital at all levels, who were having a new experience in seeing more than token numbers of minority group persons as students and beginning professionals, rather than at the lowest level of staff. Of course, the six Hampton students, who had not had this experience last summer, took part both in the introductory physiology course and the introductory clinical tutorials.

Problems with Current Student Attitudes:
On Testing

The sixteen post-junior-year premedical students represented the best of the twenty-two applicants. These applicants had all been suggested to me either by premedical advisors in their colleges or by students who had come to know me and the kind of students I was trying to encourage to apply to Cornell. They were, in other words, not at all a random sample but a selected group. Our first session on June 8th was for the purpose of orientation, reviewing what the various components of the summer program would be, since our written description of the program had not mentioned the physiology course or the introductory clinical work.

In discussing the new physiology course with them, Dr. Walter Riker admitted that he and I had not felt secure enough to introduce a course into last summer's program, because we wanted each student to have the most complete opportunity to work with his faculty sponsor on the individual research project. He also informed them that several post-doctoral fellows and young faculty people, on reading the course outline, had asked if they could sit in on the course. He had not thought that a good plan, as it would dilute the whole experience. He went on to ask the students to realize this would not only be a learning experience for them, but it would be the same for the student teachers who would often be unsure of their performance as lecturers. There were more student-teacher volunteers than sessions in the physiology seminar, but those students who had wanted to teach were identified as being available for any additional tutoring or conversation the summer students might desire.

One of the Summer Research Fellowship students asked if there would be any tests. Dr. Riker answered that we hadn't planned it that way, but perhaps it would be a good idea, inasmuch as many students feel it helps them know how they are learning and mastering the material. At this point, I entered the discussion, suggesting that I thought tests would make the course a more realistic and worthwhile experience, and recalling my own student days when very regular testing was part of it.

In retrospect, that was perhaps not a good time for

me to have entered the discussion, but I went on to say that the course, like everything else in the summer program, was all for the purpose of helping us learn more about a student's potential than might be reflected by standard test scores and grade-point averages.

The students were invited to vote on the matter of whether or not they would have a test or no test, or two tests. They voted to have two tests, one midway and one toward the end. There were a number of other points discussed, such as: who would see the exam papers, would they be graded, would they be returned to the students, would it be a take-home exam—but none of these points seemed at the time to require further discussion or vote. Dr. Riker made the point that since the course was not official in any way, either to the medical school or to their colleges, since it was not a credit course, the students should have nothing to fear but everything to gain, and that they should look at it simply as a trial run.

Four weeks later came the day of the first test. A serious number of misunderstandings became apparent. The students were given an examination in which they were to answer any three of six questions, and were asked to hand in their examination books. Immediately this was challenged by several students. They had not known that they had to sign their names to their examination books, nor had they understood the papers were to be either handed in or graded. If they were to be graded, were the students to have a chance to discuss their work with the instructor who graded it? Finally, all but one student handed in his paper, and several days later that one complied. One student had missed the examination because of a conflict in another schedule. Troubled feelings about the examination built up all during the next week. Rumors began to circulate that on the basis of one written test in physiology, a test they had been told should not be taken at all seriously, a complete decision was being made as to their acceptance into Cornell Medical College.

Dr. Riker and I were both somewhat surprised at our alleged villainy, but on reviewing our recollections of what had been said it seemed that there were grounds for misunderstanding. On reviewing the tape recording of the initial orientation meeting, I confirmed the fact that while all of us had recalled a vote to have two tests, all of us had heard a lot of other suggestions concerning which nothing had been decided, and everyone had simply assumed everything would turn out all right. It didn't, but surely the misunderstanding was general, and unintended all around.

The tests had, of course, been graded, except by one or two of the student teachers who refused to give a grade to the questions. At any rate, it seemed that everyone had passed the test anyway; and that while four of the twenty-two had done very well, and ten had done well, only six had made an average grade, and two had made a less-than-average grade. I indicated that I would, in private interviews with each student, let them know how they did if they wanted to know, and let them know on which question they could have further discussions with one of the student teachers or tutors. I decided to allow them to vote as to whether or not they should have a second test, honestly hoping they'd vote against it, but not saying it out loud. They voted against—and the result of the questionnaire is as follows (of the twenty-two ballots submitted to the students, all were returned, along with specific suggestions made by a number of students):

Response to the Questionnaire: 100%

1. In favor of a final written test to be signed and handed in to be graded: eight students.   Opposed: fourteen students.

2. In favor of having the test returned with the grade received: ten students. Opposed: three students. No opinion: nine students.

3. In favor of having correct answers returned with test and grade: eleven students. Opposed: three students. No opinion: eight students.

4. In favor of being informed of test result, compared to that of other students: four students. Opposed: nine students. No opinion: nine students.

5. In favor of the statement that written tests reflect the students' mastery of the subject, test-taking ability, and how well the subject was taught: six students. Opposed: ten students. No opinion: six students.

Further Suggestions:

Six students stated that a second test should be optional, not mandatory, and not imposed on the group by majority vote.

One student said that a final test would interfere with work on the research project papers, "which is like a final in itself, and probably a lot more important."

One student asked for clarification "of the intended purpose of examination."

Two students mentioned that to have the test results compared would encourage competition, that a final test should be only for the individual student's benefit.

" . . . Exams ought not to be used as parameters for one's ability to do work."

"In the future, testing guidelines when supposedly left to the students should be made more explicit."

"The role of testing is to stimulate and to instigate thought; . . . if testing is discontinued the

group as a whole (barring the individual) will begin to stagnate."

Many interesting things were learned from this experience. On thinking it over, we decided that it could
have been avoided had we simply presented one test,
midway, as a part of the designed course, without put-
ting the students in the position of voting on it. Naturally they were anxious and trying not to displease
anybody at the outset, and it was not really an ideal
time to ask them if they liked tests, and to stress how it
wouldn't be taken seriously. Everyone was trying hard
to be pleasant and agreeable. But by the time several
weeks had passed, our Summer Research Fellows were
already informed of the attitudes of Cornell medical
students toward tests and examinations. These attitudes
are, to put it mildly, somewhat ambivalent and at times
rejecting. The whole business about the test served as
an issue around which the Summer Research Fellows
felt not only a strong group unity and cause, but it also
cemented their feeling of fellowship with the larger
Cornell student community.

On Rapping

Perhaps never has there been so great a communication
problem between the generations, reflected in such dis-
turbed faculty-student interaction; nor so much difficulty in communication between the sexes. The communication problem between the races has at times
seemed greater in the past few years, although this may
not be so clear-cut a conclusion as it may seem (I shall
present data on this in the next chapter). But the atmosphere is sufficiently turbulent that faculty members are
timid about extending social invitations to students. It
was in such a frame of mind that one of the faculty
members (Dr. James Baxter) in the summer of 1969
asked if I thought it would be likely to be a pleasant

experience if he invited all the students, and me, to have cocktails and dinner at his home. We were able to weigh the pros and cons quite frankly, and it was perhaps easier because both of us are psychiatrists. He and his family entertained the whole group of us twice, and it was thoroughly enjoyed by all. Twice again this summer of 1970 the whole group were their guests.

Last summer at the very end of the program, Dean Buchanan had invited the ten Hampton students and two or three faculty sponsors into his office for cocktails to express his pleasure at how well the whole program had gone. This summer, even though the group was larger, twenty-two students, the Dean felt that he would make a more generous gesture. After discussing it thoroughly, we concluded that it would be a good idea to have the whole group come to a picnic on one afternoon during the next-to-last week. The picnic would be held at York Lodge, a recreational facility used during certain times by the faculty and their families—but otherwise as a recreational facility for patients. Located on Long Island Sound, it had facilities for swimming, golf, tennis, hiking, and for picnics. The students and the faculty sponsors were all to be the guests of the Dean and all the members of the Dean's staff.

Transportation was to be provided for the whole group of us to arrive there at about 3:30 P.M. and to leave at about 7:30 P.M.

One week prior to this scheduled picnic, one of the Summer Research Fellows mentioned in the course of our one-to-one interview (I had four such interviews with each student in the last four weeks of the program), that there was a lot of negative feeling about the picnic. Asked to explain, he said that some students felt that it was a patronizing gesture, that they were being treated like poor little kids from the slums who were being bussed out to the countryside for some good clean fresh air, that it was too big a production just to have a picnic. It came as a surprise but I welcomed his telling me this ahead of time, because the Dean and I most certainly intended it to be simply an occasion for friendly relaxation and fun. We would not want to have people come only out of a sense of duty. We concluded that I would meet the students as a group, just at the conclusion of their next scheduled physiology seminar, and that I would ask the group to reconsider the wisdom of the planned picnic.

When I arrived at the end of the student teacher's lecture, he had just been asked to comment on the environment at Cornell. He spent the next fifteen minutes in giving an extended answer while I listened in silence, determined to let him say everything for as long as he wished. Let me say that this was a white student, proud of being an activist, undoubtedly friendly in his intentions toward blacks, who would be certain always to take a stand which he felt would most assertively champion their cause. What he had to say reflected the standard militant extremism, but what I found distressing about his oratory was his apparent assumption that all blacks are card-carrying Black Panthers and all Puerto Ricans are Young Lords.

He said that Cornell is a racist institution, never forget it, and that even though the Fellows may feel that they've been treated well here, they should not be fooled. They are still considered to be niggers by most of the whites here, while the other whites are phony liberals who ride around in air-conditioned limousines feeling sorry for the poor blacks and Puerto Ricans. On he went to explain that the real reason Cornell and other big schools are trying to get more blacks into their school has nothing to do with altruism. It has everything to do with riots in the street, and a fear of everything being burned down, and of students who threatened to tear down this rotten government. Besides, it is only being done because a lot of government money comes to the school.

When it came my turn to speak I appeared not to be shocked, and really wasn't, because his message is fairly familiar, but I felt considerable dismay. During the following week I managed to correct only one of his more egregious errors of fact; explaining that the government, far from giving money to help bring minority group students into medical schools, has actually cut down on scholarships and loans in the past two years. Fortunately the Fellows realized that the student teacher was rapping, and they had had many experiences all over the medical school and the hospital wards and clinics without a single racial incident or slight. Everywhere they were met by friendly staff, not only medical students, willing and eager to stop what they were doing sometime to explain or teach or get to know them. Meanwhile, in their rooms in the medical dormitory during evenings they had heard and taken part in rap sessions of that kind all along, and they were quite unruffled by such talk.

I explained that I had come to find out if they wanted to have a picnic. The Fellows voted on the picnic; and since I observed that a few people didn't vote as they had told me they felt, I knew I was not making much headway. I explained that the picnic really should be called off, since at least a third seemed either not to want it, or were undecided. This wouldn't amount to a party atmosphere. It was canceled, with a sigh of relief on my part, and with a suggestion that they could suggest some other kind of affair if they wished. Two days later, twenty of the twenty-two students signed a petition stating that they wanted the picnic, and they felt that it was unfair for the whole group to be denied a good time because one or two people were unsociable and didn't want it. Quite plainly it seemed that we should forget the picnic and chalk it up to experience. The Fellows were able to accept this arrangement with understanding.

It would be easy to gain the impression that minority group students attending colleges, universities, and medical schools these days must run the gauntlet between two foes: the diehard segregationists and their would-be friends, the new breed of radical student activists who do not believe the system is capable of changing enough to serve our human needs, and do not welcome evidence of constructive or peaceful change.

But these sixteen post-junior-year students were a sturdy lot. In my judgment thirteen of them would do well in this or any medical school. They have basic common sense and judgment, a sense of direction, and a clear eye on the possibilities of career success in the field of medicine.

Cornell's Future Plans

The New York Hospital—Cornell Medical Center is requesting support this year to develop and expand a program to encourage greater numbers of minority group students to enter the fields of medicine, nursing, allied medical sciences, and the entire range of health careers. While college-level programs can be aimed specifically toward medicine as a career, high-school-level programs must be more broadly based to include other health careers. Specific contacts and collaborations have been arranged with specific schools, administrators, guidance counselors, and other agencies who have helped us to identify motivated, individual students in the ninth through twelfth grades of the New York City public school system.

Students attending the New York public schools, whether they are or are not members of minority groups, are usually the children of low-income families. It is our premise that the impoverishment of their fam-

ilies and/or their minority group membership deprives
most of these youngsters from opportunities to learn
about, or to gain the encouragement and supportive
financial aid to enter, the full variety of health careers.
Such students, if they work in medical centers at all,
usually end up by default holding only those jobs of
lowest status and remuneration. The staff of the New
York Hospital and of the Cornell University Medical
College will therefore seek and arrange new opportunities to recruit and develop more fully the interests
and abilities of students who have had little stimulus to
enter the health professions.

A Program of One-to-One Support for Especially Disadvantaged High-School Students

The previously mentioned Metropolitan Committee for
Minority Groups in Medicine consists of representatives
of the admissions offices of each of the seven New York
City medical schools. This group has met monthly to
exchange views and programs and possible approaches
to the more effective recruitment and support for minority group students interested in medical careers. One
effort of that committee during 1969 was to arrange for
a meeting which was attended by high school guidance
counselors and premedical advisors from the local area
colleges, as well as by representatives from medical
school deans' staffs. The decision was arrived at following that meeting that special efforts would be made to
support those minority group students attending high
schools who were already enrolled in specially funded
programs to encourage the college entry of potentially
able, disadvantaged high school students. These were,
in fact, the only group of students already identified,
with whom we could make easy contact.

Accordingly, the directors of the College Bound,
College Discovery—SEEK, and Aspiration Search pro-

grams were asked to forward to me the names of those graduating high school seniors who met the following qualifications: they were definitely planning to become premedical students in college; they had achieved an overall grade-point average of B; and they had been accepted into at least one college, which they were planning to enter in the fall of 1970. It developed that from all these programs we obtained a total of approximately one hundred students, which meant that each of the seven medical schools was forwarded the names of approximately fifteen of these students.

At Cornell we invited the fifteen students to visit the medical school during the spring of 1970, when they met members of our student body and faculty. It is our plan to maintain an individualized, friendly and supportive contact with these students throughout their three to four years of premedical study. It is also our plan to help the students, most of whom are attending college in the metropolitan area, to receive the friendly, supportive guidance of premedical advisors in their particular colleges. We hope to insure in whatever ways are possible that the students take the proper sequence of studies and are involved in other activities which will strengthen their success as premedical students. We also plan to make available opportunities for the students to obtain summer employment at the Cornell University Medical Center, to increase their awareness of opportunities and the challenges which are involved in the medical career.

It is our plan to remain in touch with the directors of the special high school programs for disadvantaged minority-group students, in order to receive a similar group of approximately fifteen such senior students each year. Because of the special difficulties the great majority of these students will have suffered, it is my estimate that only few of them will survive the high school years with good academic records, considering the amount of academic retardation and financial impoverishment which they must show before they are selected for these programs. Those few who complete high school and college with good performance profiles should be very highly regarded as excellent candidates for medicine.

A Program of One-to-One Support for High School Students of High Academic Potential

As a result of work during the past six to seven years, I continue to be persuaded of the importance of developing volunteer, big-brother-like programs in which minority group students of higher-than-average ability would be brought into a supportive friendship with a minority group professional adult. It is my feeling that it is possible to develop supportive friendships across social-class and racial lines, and that it is a constructive experience for which opportunities should be provided. The great majority of minority group children attending our public schools have only rarely the experience of observing minority group professionals in positions of leadership. Ideally, the high school student should have the experience of supportive and friendly contacts with college, professional school students, and professional staff members who are from his own and from other groups of origin.

In one such program, that conducted by the Provident Clinical Society of Brooklyn (for which I worked as Chairman of the Scholarship Committee), which I have discussed in an earlier chapter, thirty-two of the original thirty-six students graduated from high school and twenty-nine are now enrolled in college. Ordinarily, half of these students would have been high school drop-outs. Dr. Abraham Tauchner, Assistant Superintendent of the 16th School District of Brooklyn, and members of his guidance and counselling staff, have continued to meet with me and to discuss ways in which greater academic and professional career development could be achieved with the very talented minority group child.

These children are at risk for four reasons which are not known generally: (*1*) high-ability children are placed in (IGC) Classes for Intellectually Gifted Children, usually at some time between second and sixth grades, and in so-called (SP) Special Progress Classes in the seventh through ninth grades; (*2*) programs for these classes are almost all academically oriented, with no definite parent or family involvement with career orientation or with other relevent social needs; (*3*) when these children go on to high schools, they no longer receive any special class or designation, and not all of them even end up in an academic track or in a high school which can adequately prepare them for college work; (*4*) because they are not academically retarded, they *do not* qualify for inclusion in programs funded by HEW under the *Upward Bound Guidelines.* Guidelines for these programs exclude students who are not initially academically retarded, and who are not from extremely impoverished families.

For all children in School District 16 in 1969–1970 who were in an IGC or SP Class (a total of seven hundred and thirty-three students who completed the form), a simple form was devised providing identifying data for the child and his family, his career interests, and parents' work and career aspirations. For grades two through nine, the five highest career interest areas were: teaching (one hundred and sixty-one students), medicine (eighty-five students), nursing (seventy-seven students), science (fifty-five students), engineering (forty-four students). This shows a relatively high rate of interest in health careers.

We were particularly interested in identifying those students who would be graduating from junior high in June 1970, and who would be entering ninth or tenth grade in the fall of 1970. We had the following aims in mind: (*1*) to help assure that the student attended a high school at which he would receive academic preparation to assure his getting into a college or university which would allow him to realize his career ambitions; (*2*) particularly for students interested in medicine and nursing, to make maximal use of the resources of the Cornell Medical Center, medical and nursing students as well as staff, and to provide each student with at least one concerned and interested adult who would come to know the student and his family.

We were able to identify a total of thirty students, who will be either ninth or tenth graders, who have expressed interest in the field of medicine (eighteen) or nursing (twelve). We have also identified many students, and a smaller number of faculty in the Medical School, the Nursing School, and the Graduate School of Medical Sciences, who have expressed willingness to become acquainted with these students. I am able to arrange for these students to meet in small groups with their individual sponsors.

Many if not most of these students could make leadership contributions in the fields of medicine, medical research, nursing, or allied fields. Lacking such a program, they run a high risk of becoming drop-outs from health or professional careers.

A Medical Explorer Post

In the spring of 1970, arrangements were made with Mr. Earl Allyn, Vice-President of the Boy Scouts of America, working to develop medical exploring activity in the metropolitan area, to provide us with guidance on setting up such a post at the New York Hospital—Cornell Medical Center.

Prior experience had shown that high school juniors and seniors, boys and girls, would profit from the setting up of such Medical Explorer Posts at hospitals where they were welcomed. A standardized organizational format has been arrived at, and was followed in our case. Students volunteer to come for one or several hours a week to do volunteer work in the hospital under the individual guidance of an adult already working in the health field of the student's interest. Students also form a club which meets every other week where they learn and observe the role of the various hospital departments and fields.

We decided to select the Julia Richman High School, located only a few blocks away from our medical center. Julia Richman High School is now coeducational, draws students from all over the city, and was formerly known to have a strong program for girls interested in nursing. Currently it is estimated that about seventy percent of the student body is black or Puerto Rican.

An interest survey was conducted for students who will be in the eleventh or twelfth grade in the fall of 1970. It was found that of one hundred and eighty-three expressed career interests, thirty-seven students were interested specifically in medical careers, seventy-five in nursing, twenty-four in psychology, twenty in social work, sixteen in biological or biochemical technology, five in home economics, four in food management, one in optometry, and one in veterinary medicine.

All one hundred and eighty-three students were sent written letters of invitation to come to the medical center for their first organizational meeting. A professional advisory council for the Explorer Post was formed to provide organizational support and leadership. The first meeting was attended by one hundred and seventy Julia Richman students who enjoyed the brief program which had been prepared, heard a welcome and a description of the program, and elected their officers of

President, 1st Vice-President, 2nd Vice-President, Secretary, and Treasurer.

The second organizational meeting was held in the same place one week later, and was attended by seventy-nine Julia Richman students who handed in their applications for membership in the Explorer Post. They also saw two film strips in which was presented the great variety of health career fields. The students were introduced in person to representatives of most of the departments of the hospital, where they will be given the opportunity to do volunteer work beginning in the fall of 1970. It is anticipated that about fifty students will remain with a more or less continuing participation in the Medical Explorer Post.

Summary

We have described the process during which over a two-year period, 1968–1970, the Cornell University Medical College joined other leading medical schools of the nation in admitting greater numbers of minority group students.

In some detail we have discussed the changes in admissions policies of the seven medical schools in the New York City area, all of which previously had admitted only token numbers of minority group students, less than two percent as a rule. Of all medical freshmen who entered in 1969, minority group students comprised five percent, and the percentage of entering freshmen in 1970 had risen to eight percent.

This New York metropolitan area experience suggests that the recently suggested goal as set forth by the Task Force of the Association of American Medical Colleges is a reasonable one, and that by 1975, it is possible that minority group students will comprise twelve percent of the American medical student body.

This development sets the stage for profound

changes and improvement in the delivery of high quality medical education in this country, and to the delivery of high quality health care to the whole American
community.

Medical schools can take the initiative in estab-
lishing collaborative programs with interested faculty
and students at colleges and at the high schools to facili-
tate the early identification, supportive guidance and
other supports, to assure that the minority group student who enters medical school will compete on a comfortable level of dignity with his other classmates.

Serious oversights and blunders in policy by which
many compensatory educational programs for disadvantaged high-school and college-level students have
been identified, and programs have been suggested such
as would correct these more obvious errors.

Successful recruitment of potentially able medical
students involves not only working with college students at all levels as well as high-school level students,
but provisions also must be made to recruit for all the
health-related professions and fields. Details of the Cornell—New York Hospital Medical Center activities, as
they presently operate and are projected, are reviewed.

Despite serious communication problems which
have been recently manifest between young people and
the older generation, as specifically manifested in dis-
turbed faculty-student interaction, positive coalitions
of constructively oriented students and faculty can be
formed and can succeed in bringing out desirable institutional change.

VII

Will They Return to the Ghetto?

Introduction

In this chapter we shall attempt to answer a few of the most often asked questions on the implications for health care of the desegregation of medical education. Among these questions certainly the most popular one is: Will the black graduates return to practice medicine in the ghetto? Judging from written responses on the applications they submitted for medical school admission, for the classes entering Cornell in 1969 and 1970, respectively twenty-five and ninety-five black applicants in those two years, the overwhelming majority stated directly or indirectly that they plan to return to the ghetto, and are primarily motivated to enter medicine because their people so desperately need medical care. In further conversation with many of these students, I had no doubt that they themselves believe it would be a noble and altruistic act if they were to open up an office, presumably as a solo practitioner, and become a general practitioner in a black urban ghetto. Similar impressions were found from my conversations with other medical admissions interviewers. How is this explained? Perhaps most superficially it can be explained as part of the current black student ideology, that the student feels he is expected at least to make such a statement. It is easy to speculate further that the prospective medical student probably perceives that such statements seem to have a favorable effect on other black students who might otherwise deride his choice of a conservative field, and it might also have a favorable effect on whites who harbor either romantic liberal or segregationist feelings. My own first reaction to this phenomenon was to consider it a current fad or fashionable view, probably of a passing nature. My further thoughts were that some of them undoubtedly would return to the ghetto, particularly if they had formerly lived in all-black neighborhoods as almost all of them had, but that they would remain only so long as it took them to earn enough money from their practice to move away to a suburb or to a more desirable neighborhood in the city.

Unfortunately, segregation in medical care as in so many other aspects of American life has formed a great part of our national heritage. It is fairly safe to predict that most of the newly graduated black physicians will spend a major part of their professional career working mainly with black patients. This is the way it has always been for most black physicians. For this reason, there is no novelty in the students' pronouncement that they will return to the ghetto. It would be truly novel if greater numbers of young black physicians should migrate to all parts of the country, and to all parts of metropolitan areas, and not confine themselves so rigidly to the inner city of large urban areas.

In an earlier day, P. B. Cornely[1] pointed out that Negro physicians, although educated at Howard and Meharry presumably to take care of the health needs of the great mass of southern rural Negroes, were actually migrating to urban communities to serve the health needs of Negroes migrating to more prosperous urban communities. In precisely the same way, we can almost certainly predict that black physicians will increasingly migrate to the suburbs to care for the health needs of the more prosperous blacks who migrate to the suburbs. But we can also expect that with a gradual lowering of racial and color barriers in American life, black physicians and black patients, white physicians and white patients will not allow racial considerations to complicate their pursuit of good health care. This will be delayed by the continuation of segregated and second-class medical education for blacks for black patients only.

Judging from my own personal experience and observations as a black physician in the New York City area for twenty years or more, I have come to know, at least slightly, approximately two hundred black physicians and dentists in the area. Observations on where they live and where they practice are relevant. Very few of them, certainly under ten per cent, have their homes and offices in the middle of the most deprived parts of the black ghetto. As many as a third to a half of them have their offices in such locations, but their homes are located in more desirable neighborhoods outside the all-black ghetto neighborhood. Most of these physicians, in whatever location, have almost all black patients in their private practice, while fewer than five per cent have a majority of white patients. Private office practice continues largely to be racially segregated, but is very much a matter of the physician's personal choice.

It is not my impression, however, that the great bulk of medical practice and health care in the ghetto is dispensed from doctors' offices. It is my distinct impression that most black patients go to municipal or voluntary hospitals or clinics for medical care, and that it is the quality of care given in these facilities which determines their health outcome. Certainly this is true for the more serious or chronic diseases and disorders, those requiring the most complicated diagnostic procedures and therapeutic programs. Those of my black professional colleagues who are the most highly trained specialists spend a large part of their time in such hospital and clinic settings, and also spend part of their time in medical school teaching, research, or administration. Moreover, most of my colleagues either took part in, or had a lively interest in, the struggle of black professionals to gain appointments on the staff of these hospitals, and to obtain the admission and equal treatment of Negro patients to these public and private community institutions. As the practice of medicine has become increasingly dependent on scientific technology, it has depended more and more on the highly trained specialist staff at teaching hospitals. The solo practitioner practicing in his office in the ghetto, or in any other neighborhood, is only one small element in the medical manpower team. It would be unfortunate indeed if a disproportionately large share of the black physicians who will be graduating during the next decades had a too-limited view of their potential medical role. The most impressive instance of what I thought an unwise plan was one young man who has the potential of becoming a top medical research scientist, because of his earlier interest and a superb background in mathematics and the physical sciences, but who seriously intends to become a general practitioner in one of the New York City ghettos. For this reason we should examine more fully the issues and problems which are inherent in ghetto health-care delivery.

Racial Neighborhood Territoritality

The mass migration of Negroes from the rural South to northern urban centers from 1940 until the present time has been the single most important development in the process of the Negro's becoming a complete American citizen. Restrictions on residential areas open to Negroes led to the rapid growth of all-black central city ghettos, accompanied by a simultaneous massive migration of whites to surrounding suburban areas. As John F. Kain has pointed out, the net in-migration of southern Negroes accounted for 54 percent of the 2.7 million increase in the northern Negro population in the 1950–1960 decade alone, and now the Negro population is almost evenly divided between North and South.[2] In New York City, for example, in the 1950–1960 decade 476,000 whites left the central city, while 240,000 Negroes moved in; but in the same decade 1,777,000 whites moved to New York City's suburban ring, while only 67,000 Negroes moved to those suburbs. It is essential to bear in mind all these various directions of population movement, South to North, urban to suburban, in plans to affect ghettos as such. In 1960 the 216 metropolitan areas of the U.S. were eleven percent Negro. However, seventeen percent of their central cities was Negro and only five percent of the suburban population of these metropolitan areas was Negro. New York City in 1960 was typical of most northern metropolitan areas, with fourteen percent Negro population in its central-city area, and only three percent of Negroes in its suburban ring. This is not readily explained on socioeconomic grounds, since low-income whites have moved to suburbia in great numbers, and many middle-income Negro families remain in the central cities even though they would be able to afford homes in the suburbs.

Continuing overt and subtle racial prejudice and fear of rejection undoubtedly contribute to the slowness of many Negroes to seek better housing, schools, jobs, and other strong neighborhood resources in the suburbs. Jack Rothman has described the process by which real estate agents, banks, and lending institutions, advertising in a certain way in the Negro press, manage to create and maintain ghetto neighborhoods.[3] These same groups "willingly inject lower-class and 'problematic' elements into an evolving middle-class Negro or inter-racial community, thus thwarting the efforts of colored teachers, doctors, lawyers and businessmen to enjoy the benefits of a reasonable standard of community living for themselves and their children" (Rothman). The chief means by which this is done is to sell a home to a client who cannot afford it, making it necessary to complete a series of devious financing deals, with the result that the would-be owner must overcrowd the home to gain enough income to pay for his mortgages. What is clearly indicated is a program to bring about managed suburban neighborhood integration as Anthony Downs suggests,[4] with a deliberate plan of preserving a middle-class neighborhood life-style which is not in essence the exclusive property of any single racial group or skin color. Two out of three Negroes prefer living in a racially integrated residential area, but they do not usually cite superior neighborhood facilities as the reason; rather they wish to have the "psychological effect of liberation from the ghetto" and the desire to improve the image of Negroes held by whites. Racially integrated schooling and integrated employment are favored by margins of seven to one, but the margin favoring integrated housing drops to three to one (Brink and Harris).[5] It is doubtful that this great a proportion of Negroes is expressing self-segregation attitudes so much as anticipatory rejection.

White attitudes toward Negroes have been reviewed by Paul B. Sheatsley in the twenty-year period from 1942 to 1963.[6] In 1942, not one American white in three approved of integrated schools. Only two percent of white southerners favored racially integrated schools, but a majority of white northerners also opposed them. White attitudes shifted to a majority support for integration following the 1954 Supreme Court ruling against the "separate but equal" doctrine. By 1956, eleven percent of whites in the South and most whites in the North favored it, so that on a nationwide basis it could be said that half the white population favored integrated schools. There were continued advances until 1963, when thirty-four percent of the white South said white and Negro students should go to the same schools; seventy-three percent of the white North agreed, and the nationwide figure was sixty-three percent. These trends have been maintained even during the racial separatist atmosphere of the past few years. By mid-1965, fifty-five percent of southern whites favored integrated schools. From the end of 1963 to the middle of 1965 was a period of relatively rapid change of opinion among whites in the South; the number who would not object to a Negro neighbor changed from fifty-one percent to sixty-six percent. Of even greater interest was the observation that among southern whites whose children had actually attended school with Negroes, seventy-four percent said that Negroes and whites should attend the same schools, while only forty-eight percent held that belief if their children had not had the actual experience. All these findings point to the obvious conclusions that there has been a steady and marked increase within the past decade in the number of whites in the North and the South who favor neighborhood and school integration, and that attitudes toward integration are more positive where it has actually been experienced by whites. It is all the more remarkable that slogans persist to the effect that integration has been tried and failed; integration is dead; nobody is in favor of integration, and so forth. As Sheatsley concludes, "As higher proportions of the nation's youth go on to college, as higher proportions enter white-collar and professional rather than farm or production employment, and as (and if) family income levels continue to rise, we may reasonably expect the

long-term trend in white attitudes toward acceptance
of racial integration not only to continue but even to
accelerate."

Ghetto Problems and Plans

There are two rival schools of thought today concerning
what should be done to solve the problems of persons
who live in our large all-black urban ghettoes. One
school maintains that segregation will be with us for a
long time, that it will increase, that racial separatism is
desirable, that separation will allow the black community to become strong and unified and in a better position
to become integrated with other Americans later on.
This school of thought accepts the fact of segregation
and favors improving, renewing, rebuilding, and some
would say "gilding" the ghetto. Measures are taken to
encourage firms to locate in the ghetto, to foster black-
owned businesses, to involve the black community in
rehabilitating and renewing their houses, and generally
to gain black control over all public as well as private
agencies which operate in the ghetto. The more extreme
proponents of this view, the militant black separatists,
do not have the aim of ever becoming part of a racially
integrated American society. Rather they look forward
to becoming a separate black nation within a white
nation. Because racial separation has had so long a role
in American life, it is not surprising that this school of
thought would gain support from conservatives, from
radical militants of both races, as well as from tired and
not-too-well-informed liberals.

The second school of thought, presented by John
F. Kain and Joseph J. Persky, which has been the traditional position of militant civil rights Negro leadership
for at least a hundred and fifty years, holds that urban
Negroes, and the enlightened American citizenry as a
whole, should be unwilling to accept the permanence
of central ghettos or of racial separatism in neighbor-

hoods, housing, schools, or other aspects of community life.[7] Massive programs to strengthen the ghetto by developing all-black plans to build schools, homes, business firms to employ blacks, and a whole set of specifically black health, education, and welfare services will only delay the full entry of American blacks into first-class American citizenship. In other words, only by dispersal or destruction of the ghetto can the blacks currently confined there be freed to develop as strong individuals and families.

Moreover the plans to strengthen the black ghetto in the North would probably have unanticipated and untoward effects, as Kain and Persky have pointed out. Unless a simultaneous and rapid program were developed to strengthen and make it more attractive for Negroes to remain in the rural South, artificially improved northern ghettos would receive an unmanageable influx of uneducated and otherwise handicapped blacks who would seriously disrupt such plans. The fundamental argument, however, is that ghettos are artificially contrived and externally controlled. Such neighborhoods should and can be prevented from their destructive growth. The existence of suburbs and ghettos are opposite sides of a single coin, directly and indirectly responsible for the failure of urban renewal, the crisis in central-city finance, the urban transportation crisis, Negro unemployment and welfare, and the failure of public education. Even if the ghettos were simply dispersed to the suburbs, with small ghetto enclaves scattered throughout them, this would immediately bring to blacks better housing, jobs, and schools, and at only a fraction of the cost of massive ghetto-gilding programs.

For a fuller presentation of ghetto problems, Kenneth Clark has provided a detailed description of Harlem in New York City.[8] In reviewing the demography of Central Harlem, he takes up first its physical characteristics—its space, housing, and facilities—and then its population and socioeconomic characteristics. There is no necessity for me to detail the overcrowding and the lack of play space for children, which in part contribute to the high accidental-death rate of youngsters from motor vehicles. The deteriorated and dilapidated housing, owned by absentee landlords, presents serious hazards. With the inadequate heating systems in these houses, it is no wonder that the incidence of fires is very high. It should also be noted that despite superficial appearances, Harlem has a severe transportation problem. Subway and bus stops are inconveniently located. Taxis, especially, are reluctant to bring passengers into or out of Harlem after dark, and sometimes even during daylight hours, because of the fear of violence or robbery. Facilities are severely lacking, there being few large businesses providing employment within walking distance. Most small businesses are owned by whites. The "property, apartment houses, stores, businesses, bars, concessions, and theatres are for the most part owned by individuals who reside outside the community and who take their profits outside the community. Negroes are only involved in the more marginal businesses like beauty parlors, barber shops, and the most tenuous of grocery and candy stores. Even the numbers racket, which is such a pervasive and indestructible part of Harlem economy, is not controlled by Harlem's residents." Both the numbers racket and the narcotics traffic (Negroes comprise half the heroin addicts in the city) are controlled by the white crime syndicate. The police are widely known to be involved in accepting, even demanding, payoffs to allow numerous small Negro operations to run small gambling games and other illegal enterprises catering to exotic or perverted tastes.

All the foregoing description still fails to give the reader an impression of what it is like to live in a ghetto neighborhood. It means usually not being able to find a grocery well stocked with a wide choice of fairly priced food, not being able to find a choice of adequate restaurants, nor a five-and-dime store, nor any range or variety of shops, nor a movie theater in which one feels comfortable, nor newspapers or magazines. Most of all, there is the feeling of not being safe after dark, the psychological effect of knowing that the homicide rate in Harlem is six times the rate for the city as a whole; that the narcotics addiction rate is ten times the general city rate; that the police, though present in greater numbers than in most neighborhoods, are not generally thought to be too helpful.

Clark also found that the Harlem population did not have as many newcomers from the South as is commonly supposed; in fact only four percent of its residents were recent migrants from the South. There was, however, a major out-migration of the 21-to-44 age group. "These people are at the peak of their years of production, more responsive to changes in employment opportunities, and involved in raising families. They also tend to be the most active segment of the community with respect to participation in social and civic affairs. It is reasonable to conclude that, during the decade of the 1950's, Central Harlem thus lost a considerable part of its actual and potential leadership."

The median income for families and unrelated individuals in Central Harlem is $3,480, as compared to $5,103 for all residents of New York City. Half of all Central Harlem families earn under $4,000, compared to a quarter of New Yorkers as a whole. Whereas one in about six New York City families earned more than $10,000, only one in twenty-five Central Harlem families earned that amount. Immediately one is confronted with the major reason, lack of money, that the lifestyle of the community reflects so much frustrated rage or apathetic despair. Add to this the fact that an extraordinarily high proportion of young people in this area do not live with both parents. Half of the young people under eighteen live with only one parent or with no parent, and only half (as contrasted with eighty-three percent city-wide) live with both parents. This is a reflection of the high rate of one-parent households and the high rate of separation among parents. It should also be noted that in the 21-to-44 age group, it is the family with two parents which is more likely to leave Harlem to move to a better neighborhood, leaving behind the one-parent families.

Further analysis revealed that in Central Harlem unemployment as such was not as highly correlated with various indices of social pathology as had been anticipated, suggesting that the problem was one of low pay and low status associated with their jobs. It was much clearer that low levels of formal schooling, low family income, and lack of parental presence in the families were associated with the higher health district indices of social pathology (such indices being the juvenile delinquency rate, proportion of families receiving aid to dependent children, venereal disease rate, and homicide rate). Only low correlations were found for overcrowded or unsound housing, male unemployment, and recent migration from the South.[8]

Ghetto Health Care

The National Advisory Commission on Civil Disorders stated, "The residents of the racial ghetto are significantly less healthy than most other Americans. They suffer from higher mortality rates, higher incidence of major diseases, and lower availability and utilization of medical services. They also experience higher admission rates to mental hospitals."[9] Herbert M. Morais, citing a 1967 White House report on black ghetto life, comments on the obvious association between poverty and lack of medical care, as such, as well as the fact of improper diets, inadequate shelter and clothing and unsanitary living conditions which also seriously interfere with health care. He adds, "The life expectancy of non-whites is lower in all adult age groups. Maternal and infant mortality rates are declining for all races, but remain much higher among non-whites; four times greater in maternal deaths and twice as high in infant mortality. Non-whites at all income levels pay fewer visits to doctors and dentists and are more likely to be treated in clinics. They suffer more disabling and chronic illnesses."[10]

The Medicare and Medicaid health programs dating from 1965, and the Office of Economic Opportunities neighborhood health units from 1966 represent federal efforts to bring greater health care to the ghetto, but close observation does not reveal a significant impact up to now. Severe shortages in health manpower, rapidly spiraling costs of all components of health service, fiscal and bookkeeping delays, and the overt and subtle opposition to these programs from large segments of organized medicine have all rendered these efforts of little effect. Even more fatal is the obvious fact that effective health care simply cannot be delivered in an environment of rampant social deprivation and pathology, certainly not without massive supportive social welfare services, family services, education, job training and child care services, and housing services.

We have also observed that those ghetto dwellers who are most achievement-oriented, young adults who marry and have children and are employed, tend to move away to more desirable neighborhoods or to the suburbs. If we are to assume that future black physicians will wish primarily to have practices with black patients, those would be the families most likely to use and to be able to pay for their services. However, even non-white families with incomes of $10,000 a year or more spend less than comparable white families for health care. Their total yearly medical expenditure was only $133 compared to $179 per person in the white

family. Both groups spent $34 per person per year
(1962) for hospitals; non-whites spent $50 for doctors
compared to $61 for whites; non-whites spent $19 for
dentists compared to $37 for whites; non-whites spent
$23 for medicine compared to $31 for whites. Total non-
white medical expenditure was on the average only 74.3
percent of white expenditures (NACCD 1968). There
is, therefore, a financial sacrifice involved in the decision to have an exclusively Negro clientele. This is of
some practical importance in view of the fact that the
black physician or dentist in the New York City area, for
example, can control the racial balance of his practice
almost predictably simply by selecting the area in which
to locate his office. This has been true for at least the
past two decades.

Just as the black physician is free to determine the
extent to which he will have a racially integrated practice, the same freedom holds for the prospective Negro
patient, who is free to select his physician without regard to race. Andrew F. Brimmer has discussed the fact
that segregation served the function of providing a pro-
tective tariff for the Negro businessman.[11] As desegregation becomes an increasing feature of American life,
this will cause serious problems for Negro businessmen
who will be unable to compete as equals with other businessmen for Negro or white clients. During the 1950's
and 1960's the numbers of Negro businesses in several
key areas declined, especially self-employed single en-
trepreneurs in sanitary services, transportation, furniture, hardware, and building materials. The trend
toward the use of more sophisticated equipment, such
as refrigerator trucks and other specialty vehicles, as an
example, required more capital than most Negro truck-
ers could raise. Generally, small retailers, regardless of
race, are unable to withstand competition from super-
markets and discount chains. Negro hotel owners have
lost business now that Negro travelers are free to seek

lodging accommodations in the general marketplace. Every one of these trends applies directly to the future Negro physician practitioner. He will less and less be able to depend upon a captive black clientele.

Increasingly, opportunities are opening up for Negro managers in the corporate business community, to fulfill real functions and not only to satisfy certain "image-making" or legal requirements. Opportunities will develop for Negroes in the health industry, which is rapidly becoming one of the major industries in the country. Past discrimination has so severely limited educational and employment aspirations, the educational curriculum of most southern Negro colleges has been so archaic, and the pattern of occupational choice has been so much away from business administration or technical areas, that recruitment of black business managers will understandably be difficult. This kind of work will appeal to some future black physicians, who will have interests in hospital and health service administration. Brimmer's 1966 recommendations on the need of black businessmen to prepare themselves so that they will become competitively successful with others in an integrated society seem far sounder in my opinion than efforts to build a separate sheltered black economy within the ghetto.

Even the neighborhood health clinics funded by OEO, and endorsed by the National Medical Association, incurred some criticism from that association of black physicians. Morais reported that in 1968 NMA voiced its concern that medical schools wanted to play too great a role in supervising the clinic staff, that the clinics were not advising patients of their right to use private physicians or other providers under Medicaid, and that patients were being provided special travel allowances and baby-sitting services to go to the clinic, but not to a private physician's office. The general complaint was that local physicians, as well as local residents, were not sufficiently in charge of planning the health service. It is obvious that the best interests of patients might not coincide with the best interests of individual physicians viewing themselves as rivals of the neighborhood clinic. Much careful thought and planning must be given in the future to the role of private practitioners, groups, clinics, hospital outpatient departments, and other such providers of health care, all of whom are able to collect public funds for health services they claim to deliver to impoverished people in the ghetto. The patient's interests are likely to be the first to suffer in such a tangled struggle for control. This is only another reason that future black physicians would be well advised to plan not only to become individual practitioners and group practitioners. They should also plan to pursue careers in public health and medical administration; they should seek positions of influence within health agencies responsible for governmental standardsetting and funding of health services at city, state, and federal levels. They should help remove the color barrier completely from the practice of medicine, for good patient care and health maintenance is only hampered by prejudiced preoccupations with racial identity.

Summary

It is to be hoped that the increased numbers of black physicians who will be receiving superior educational preparations for their successful careers as physicians will be utilized as physicians for the whole American community, and will not be encouraged to limit their work to black patients only. With increasing desegregation in many areas of American life, and an increasing receptivity to a racially integrated society, it is most unlikely that black and white health-care systems and markets can be maintained, even if racist extremists attempt to keep these segregated systems artificially intact.

Black physicians will be inclined not to locate exclusively in ghetto areas; many will also live and work in the surrounding suburbs. Others will primarily pursue careers in public health, medical administration, research, teaching, and consultation to a broad range of public and private health-care agencies.

Ghetto health-care problems, like all other serious ghetto problems, can be approached either by an attitude of attempting to enrich the total life experience within such pathological neighborhoods or by ghetto-dispersal approaches which would redistribute the ghetto and suburban populations into a single community system.

The severe shortage not only of physicians but of every category of health workers, paralleled by similar shortages in the fields of education, social services, business and technology, will provide the most powerful force toward further removal of color barriers to manpower development and to the design of a more effective national system of health-care delivery.

Notes

CHAPTER I

1. Boas, Franz, *Race and Democratic Society,* New York: J. J. Augustin Publisher, 1945.

2. Childe, V. Gordon, *Man Makes Himself* (A Mentor Book), New York and Toronto: The New American Library, Inc., 1951.

3. Franklin, John Hope, *From Slavery to Freedom,* New York: Alfred A. Knopf, 1950, Chapters 1, 2, and 3.

4. Bennett, Lerone, Jr., *Before the Mayflower: A History of the Negro in America 1619–1964,* Chicago: Johnson Publishing Company, 1962.

5. Myrdal, Gunnar, *An American Dilemma,* New York and London: Harper and Brothers Publishers, 1944.

6. Morais, Herbert M., *The History of the Negro in Medicine,* A Volume of The International Library of Negro Life and History, New York and Washington: Publishers Company, Inc., 1967. Revised edition 1969.

7. Ginsberg, Eli and Eichner, Alfred S., *The Troublesome Presence,* "American Democracy and The Negro," New York: The Free Press of Glencoe, Collier-Macmillan Limited, 1964.

8. Leikind, Morris C., "Colonial Epidemic Diseases," *Ciba Symposia,* Vol. 1: 372–378, 1940.

9. Jordan, Winthrop D., *White Over Black,* "American Attitudes Toward The Negro, 1550–1812," Chapel Hill: The University of North Carolina Press, 1968.

10. Woodward, C. Vann, *The Strange Career of Jim Crow,* second revised edition, New York: Oxford University Press, 1966.

11. Bousefield, M. O., "An Account of Physicians of Color in The United States," *Bulletin of The History of Medicine* 17:61–84, 1945.

12. Johnson, Jr., Leonard, "History of the Education of Negro Physicians," *The Journal of Medical Education* 42:439–46, 1967.

13. Cobb, W. Montague, "Howard, Meharry, and Separate Professional Education," *Bulletin of the Medico-Chirurgical Society of The District of Columbia, Inc.* 4:3–9, 1947.

14. Cobb, W. Montague, *Medical Care and the Plight of the Negro*, New York: Published by The National Association for The Advancement of Colored People, 1947.

15. *The Negro Handbook*, compiled by the editors of *Ebony*, Chicago: Johnson Publishing Company, 1966.

16. Haughton, James G., "Government's Role in Health Care Past, Present and Future," *Journal of the National Medical Association* 60:87–91, 1968.

CHAPTER II

1. Dove, Dennis B., *A Fact Sheet of Data on the Educational Process Leading to the M.D. Degree As It Relates to Black Americans*, Washington, D.C.: Association of American Medical Colleges, February 4, 1970 (private distribution).

2. Editorial: "Undergraduate Origins of Medical Students," *New York State Journal of Medicine*, October 15, 1969, p. 2645.

3. Reitzes, Dietrich C., *Negroes in Medicine*, Boston, 1958.

4. Crowley, A. E. and Nicholson, H. C., "Negro Enrollment in Medical Schools," *Journal of the American Medical Association* 210:96–100, October 6, 1969.

5. Bulletin: *Minority Student Opportunities in United States Medical Schools*, 1969–1970, June 1969, AAMC Publication.

6. Cogan, Lee, *Negroes for Medicine* (Report of a Macy Conference), Baltimore, 1968; also, *Macy Foundation Report for the Year 1967*, New York, 1968.

7. Editorial: "Schools Are Changing," *Modern Medicine* ("Medical Scene" Section), January 27, 1969, p. 51.

8. Nelson, Bernard W., Project Director, *Report of the Association of American Medical Colleges Task Force to the Inter-Association Committee on Expanding Educational Opportunities in Medicine for Blacks and Other Minority Group Studies*, Washington, D.C.: Association of American Medical Colleges, April 22, 1970.

9. Education Number: "Medical Education in The United States," *JAMA* 210:1455–1582, November 24, 1969.

10. Dorman, Gerald D., "Manpower and Education," *Physicians and Surgeons Quarterly*, Columbia University, College of Physicians and Surgeons, Vol. XIV, Winter 1969, p. 6.

11. Congress on Medical Education, Osteopathy and Medicine: Sodeman, W., "Undergraduate Education;" Nunemaker, J., "Graduate Education;" Roth, R., "Licensure and Certification," *JAMA* 209:85–96, July 7, 1969.

12. Cobb, Montague, *Medical Care and the Plight of the Negro*, New York, 1947.

13. Research Section of The Division of Manpower, Research and Development: "Representation of Minority Groups Among Psychiatric Residents," *Registry of Black Psychiatric Residents*, Washington, D.C.: American Psychiatric Association, January 1970.

14. Haynes, M. A., "Distribution of Black Physicians in the United States, 1967," *JAMA* 210:93–95, October 6, 1969.

15. Cornely, P. B., "Distribution of Negro Physicians in The United States in 1942," *JAMA* 124:826–830, 1944.

CHAPTER III

1. Plaut, R. L., *Blueprint for Talent Searching*, New York: National Scholarship Service and Fund for Negro Students, 1957.

2. Editorial: "Some Facts of Medical Life," (Comment on Report of The New York State Advisory Committee to the U.S. Commission on Civil Rights), *The New York Post*, May 24, 1964.

3. *The Negro Handbook*, compiled by the editors of *Ebony*, Chicago, 1966.

4. Curtis, James L., "A Plan to Promote Professional Careers for Negroes," *Journal of the National Medical Association* 57:168-172, 1965.

5. O'Connell, Marie and Rosen, Sidney of the Guidance Counseling Staff, District 16, New York City Board of Education, Personal Communication.

6. Davidson, Helen H. and Greenberg, Judith W., *Traits of School Achievers from a Deprived Background, a part of The Research Studies Series*, New York, 1967.

7. *1970–71 Upward Bound Guidelines*, An Office of Education Program Administration Manual, U.S. Department of Health, Education, and Welfare, Office of Education, November 1969.

8. Lopate, Carol, *The College Readiness Program: A Program for Third World Students at the College of San Mateo, California*, New York: Columbia University, ERIC Information Retrieval Center on The Disadvantaged, 1969.

9. Clark, Kenneth, "No-Nonsense Approach to Slum Schools," *Wall Street Journal* Editorial Page Article, December 26, 1969.

10. Coleman, James S., in *Equal Educational Opportunity,* an expansion of the Winter 1968 Special Issue of *The Harvard Educational Review,* Cambridge, Massachusetts, 1969.

CHAPTER IV

1. This faculty committee was composed of Dr. Robert F. Pitts, Professor of Physiology; Dr. Walsh McDermott, Professor of Public Health; Dr. Walter F. Riker, Jr., Professor of Pharmacology.

2. This committee of students was composed of Mr. Robert Robinson, Class of '71, and Mr. Jeffrey Gingold, Class of '71, who were responsible for bringing in a written report; and others.

3. Robinson, Robert, "CUMC Seeks Disadvantaged Students," *Synapse,* Winter 1969 Issue (A Cornell Medical Student Publication).

4. Frazier, E. Franklin, *The Negro in the United States,* New York, 1949.

5. Rainwater, Lee and Yancey, William L., *The Moynihan Report and The Politics of Controversy,* Cambridge, Massachusetts, 1967.

6. Frazier, E. Franklin, *Black Bourgeoisie,* New York, 1957.

7. Most of the issues discussed here were reviewed comprehensively in *Preparation for The Study of Medicine,* Page, Robert G. and Littlemeyer, Mary H., Editors, Chicago, 1969.

CHAPTER V

1. *New York Post,* Editorial Page, May 24, 1964.

2. Bulletin: *Minority Student Opportunities in United States Medical Schools, 1969–1970,* AAMC Publication, June, 1969.

3. Reitzes, Dietrich, *Negroes in Medicine,* Boston, 1958.

4. Cobb, W. Montague, "Howard, Meharry, and Separate Professional Education," *Bulletin of the Medico-Chirurgical Society of The District of Columbia, Inc.* 4:3–9, 1947.

CHAPTER VII

1. Cornely, P. B., "Distribution of Negro Physicians in the United States in 1942," *Journal of the American Medical Association* 124:826–830, 1944.

2. Kain, John F. (editor), *Race and Poverty,* "The Economics of Discrimination," Englewood Cliffs, New Jersey, 1969. Editor's Introductory Chapter.

3. Rothman, Jack, "The Ghetto Makers," *The Nation,* 193, No. 10, October 7, 1961, pp 222-225. Also excerpted and reprinted in Kain, *op. cit.*

4. Downs, Anthony, "Alternative Futures for the American Ghetto," *Daedalus,* 97, No. 4 of the Proceedings of The American Academy of Arts and Sciences, Fall 1968. "The Conscience of the City," pp. 1331–1378.

5. Brink, William and Harris, Louis, "Breaking the Vicious Circle," *The Negro Revolution in America,* New York, 1964, pp. 157–61. Also reprinted in Kain, *op. cit.*

6. Sheatsley, Paul B., "White Attitudes toward the Negro," *Daedalus: The Negro American,* 95, No. 1, Winter 1966, pp. 217–38.

7. Kain, John F. (Editor) and Persky, Joseph J., "Alternatives to the Gilded Ghetto," *The Public Interest,* No. 14, Winter 1969, pp. 74–87. Exerpted and reprinted in Kain, *op. cit.*

8. Clark, Kenneth (Director of the Study), *Youth in the Ghetto:* "A Study of The Consequences of Powerlessness and A Blueprint for Change," New York: Harlem Youth Opportunities Unlimited, Inc., 1964.

9. *Report of the National Advisory Commission on Civil Disorders,* New York, 1968.

10. Morais, Herbert M., *The History of the Negro in Medicine,* New York, 1969.

11. Brimmer, Andrew F., "The Negro in the National Economy," *The American Negro Reference Book,* Edited by Davis, John P., Englewood Cliffs, New Jersey, 1966. Also reprinted in Kain, *op. cit.*